# Queer Counselling and Narrative Practice

edited by
**David Denborough**

Many of the papers that appear in this book have been previously published in the *Dulwich Centre Journal* or *Gecko: a journal of deconstruction and narrative ideas in therapeutic practice*.

**Dulwich Centre Publications**
ADELAIDE, SOUTH AUSTRALIA

ISBN 0 9577929 6 4


**Dulwich Centre Publications**
Hutt St PO Box 7192
Adelaide 5000, South Australia
phone (61-8) 8223 3966, fax (61-8) 8232 4441
email: dcp@senet.com.au
website: www.dulwichcentre.com.au

Printed and manufactured by
Graphic Print Group, Richmond, South Australia.

# Contents

# Contents (cont'd)

## Part Three: Talking amongst ourselves



## Part Four: Therapy & lesbian lives



## Part Five: Therapeutic work with gay men



## Part Six: Bisexual experience

# *Contents* (cont'd)

## *Part Seven:* **Transgender/bi-gender experience – issues for therapists**



## *Part Eight:* **Complexities of culture, sexuality and spirituality**

# A note from the Editor

Dear Reader,

It is with delight that this book is being sent out into the world.

Each paper included here has been created from the lived experience of the authors. Every turn of phrase has been shaped by conversations, relationships, lovers, friends, colleagues, books …

These writings have been crafted with an audience of therapists, health workers, healers in mind. Some of the pieces are about direct therapeutic practice, others sketch broader landscapes, and all are of relevance to those who listen to people as they tell the stories of their lives.

For those of us whose sexual identities flourish outside the norms of heterosexual desire, and for those who are demonstrating how gendered identities are more fluid than we were led to believe, this book is a celebration of insider knowledge. But it is also much more.

The writings in this book represent a small part of a broader transformation that is occurring within the health professions. Lesbian, gay, bisexual, trans- and bi-gendered experience is disrupting the very assumptions upon which these professions are built. The boundaries of nuclear family life are dissolving and the taken-for-granted is being replaced with the unexpected. What a joy I believe this to be.

If this book was to be dedicated, it would be to future generations:

> 'May you recognise yourself in these stories. May they offer company as you celebrate your desires, your chosen love relationships, and your families, whatever shape they may take.'

With love,.
david d.

PS: The layout work for this book was done by Jane Hales. Thanks the janey!
PPS: Many of the papers in this book have previously appeared in journals by Dulwich Centre Publications. These details are provided at the back of this book, along with information about all the contributors.

# PART ONE

# *Creating families of our own*

The writings that follow, celebrate the creation of families by lesbian, gay and bisexual people and their children and loved ones. As described in these papers, for many queer people, the creation of family involves deliberate, political and loving acts. Family can be understood as a verb not a noun.

Many of the papers in this section were originally spoken at a narrative therapy and community work conference in Adelaide. The contributors are from the US, Australia and the UK.

To begin, Ann Hartman and Joan Laird, two highly respected lesbian family therapists in the US, describe how so much has changed in their lifetimes. As they describe it, in North America and especially in Massachusetts where they live, it's a 'new world' for lesbian and gay families.

# 1

# It's a new world

by

Ann Hartman & Joan Laird

***Joan:*** Our intimate extended family, spanning two homes about 40 minutes apart, consists of Ann and me, a tall, slim absolutely zany black standard poodle named Hilary, a white slightly more sedate standard poodle named Madelaine, and two handsome gentleman cats, Alfred North Whitefoot and Angus McTaggart. In a house across the valley live our son Duncan, our daughter-in-law Meg, and two scrumptious grandchildren, Hannah, almost 6 and Julian, 2½.

***Ann:*** In so many ways it's a new world for gay and lesbian people now. In the States, at least, and especially in the area of Massachusetts where we live, the last decade or two have seen so many changes that once I would not have imagined. I never knew a lesbian when I was growing up. I remember as a teenager sneaking into a drug store, hiding behind a pile of books and looking at the book 'The Well of Loneliness' which was for many people my age their only experience of lesbianism.

It was one of the first books about being lesbian and, like all the early books, it focused only on tragedy. I'll never forget the first time I walked into a gay bar and saw a room full of people like me. I was 23 years old and had always had the lonely and isolating experience of being 'the only one'.

Throughout most of my life I was totally underground. I didn't lie, nor did I pretend I had boyfriends, but it was a case of 'don't ask don't tell'. You must remember that I grew up before Stonewall. I was a middle-aged woman before lesbians, gays and transgender people in the Stonewall bar in New York fought back against police brutality and discrimination and sparked the gay liberation movement. The oppression that lesbians and gays grew up with before Stonewall was indescribable – much of it frightening. Furthermore, we had no language for this oppression, and nowhere to turn for protection. We had no language to describe our own lives and loves.

Joan and I have been together for 36 years and, for the first decades of our relationship, we did not use the 'L' word. Although we always went places together and indeed I insisted that Joan be invited to any social event that I was to be a part of, not being able to speak openly about our lives was very restrictive. It often meant that authentic conversations weren't available in our social network which almost exclusively consisted of heterosexual couples and their children. It meant that we could talk with others about work, homemaking, gardening, and children, but very little about our relationship could ever be shared.

The attitudes of the day towards lesbianism had real effects within our household. In the early years of our relationship, there was always the possibility that Joan's son, Duncan, would be taken from her. Joan's ex-husband, Duncan's father, often threatened to claim custody of Duncan. Since we knew other lesbians who had lost their children, we were very cautious and silent about our relationship, even with Duncan. We didn't want him to know something he couldn't tell his father, to have to carry this secret. To be honest, though, the fear in relation to losing custody was only one of the reasons that we never spoke to Duncan about the truth of our lives. Another was my own uneasiness and shame. Most people who grew up gay or lesbian in the years before Stonewall grew up with self narratives constituted from the heterosexist and hostile world around them. I think that was one of the major reasons that I never talked openly with Duncan. We were truly worried about the custody issue but I was also so used to aspects of my life simply not being talked about. So we did not speak to Duncan. He grew up with this secret from the time he was 18 months old until he was 19. It's difficult to know just what the costs of that silence may have been.

***Joan:*** In recent years I've learned to be more forgiving of myself about this. There is now considerable analysis of the historical and social context of the 1950s and the 1960s, which has offered me a better understanding of myself. The 1950s, in the US, was the most oppressive of times for many people. Gay and lesbian people were at risk of exposure, loss of jobs, public humiliation, and so on, just as was anyone suspected of being a Communist. McCarthyism contaminated the country. I went to an all-women's college in the 1950s that was supposed to be a hotbed of lesbianism. It was so underground I never even heard the word while I was there and certainly never met one!

I was a product of the 1950s. My parents were anxious the day after graduation that I wasn't yet married. It was a paradoxical time – women would go to college with great but undefined hopes for the future, and their families would sacrifice a great deal to send them there. But the purpose, overt or covert, was often to find a husband from a better social class – to ensure a more privileged life. I remember my roommates and I sitting around endlessly reading brides' magazines, talking about our hopes and our hope chests. What a dreadful time!

In the 1940s, when Ann was in college, it was quite different for women. It was wartime, and women were needed in the armed forces, in the factories, to perform public roles many had never performed before. It was a totally different scenario. By the 1950s the social discourse had changed to prescribe that women should not be taking jobs away from men. Instead, women were to dedicate their lives to rearing perfect children and maintaining perfect homes, domestic engineers. And that was the role I had been playing shortly before I met Ann. I had been busy being the perfect 1950s housewife. My husband and I had a demanding family business together. I worked as hard as he did in the business, but when we came home my day was just starting while his was ending. I was a 'second shift' housewife, although the discourse, for white middle-class women at least, suggested that their public work or earned income was not making a real contribution to the household. As I look back on those years, I realise that I just got more and more tired and more and more resentful. I was thirty when I finally left and Duncan, my son, was about 16 months old.

I temporarily moved in with my parents. My mother had been working as the bookkeeper for a mental health clinic in which Ann was the executive. When I asked my mother, 'Okay, what do I do now?' my mother said 'Well, we'll invite Ann Hartman over to dinner. She'll tell you what to do.'

My mother was in awe of Ann. She kept describing Ann as 'brilliant' and as a 'character'. (Little did she know just what a brilliant character Ann was!) So we did invite Ann over to dinner and Ann did indeed tell me what to do with my life! She suggested that I should become a social worker. But I also needed to earn money right away and so she suggested I come and assist her in the mental health clinic and, oh yes, I might like to come visit her summer place.

Ann had a condominium on Fire Island by the ocean, and she would invite me there for weekends. I would take Duncan in a little basket and go over on the ferry. There were always about 6 or 7 other people there and all I knew was that they knew something I didn't. I went around asking them stupid questions like 'Have you been married? Are you in a relationship with anyone?' And they were all rolling their eyes wondering where on earth Ann had found this one. I knew something was going on but I couldn't figure it out. Even as I watched all the men in their well-filled bikinis at Cherry Grove, which was the centre of gay life on the east coast, it didn't register. I just began to get more anxious.

***Ann:*** With good reason!

***Joan:*** One night I wanted to reciprocate Ann's generosity and so I bought theatre tickets and invited her to accompany me to New York for dinner and the theatre. Afterwards when we stopped in the village for coffee, Ann kept taking my arm as we crossed the street and I began to feel like I was on a date. I began to feel conspicuous and anxious, but I still didn't understand. Then Ann asked if I'd ever seen the new Verrazano Bridge which had been built over the gateway to New York harbour and I said no. She asked if I would like to see it and I said yes. Ann paid the toll and as we started to drive over this bridge, I had the strangest sensation. I knew I was never going to come back again, that she was taking me somewhere. I've been afraid of heights ever since!

In some ways I was right. One night when I was visiting out on Fire Island, and we were sleeping in separate beds, Ann reached over and gently laid her hand on my head. In some terror, I asked, 'What are you doing?', followed up with a very formal speech in which I said to Ann that I liked her very much but I just was not that sort of woman.

***Ann:*** I said that I was that sort of woman and that I had been all of my life.

***Joan:*** The next night I wouldn't go in the bedroom. I had the first anxiety attack I'd ever had. I just sat in a chair in the middle of summer in the living room and grew colder. I kept collecting blankets but the cold would not go away. Ann was in bed and the baby had gone to sleep as I just sat there for hours wrapped up in blankets, shaking and shaking. And then finally, I got up and went into the bedroom and Ann tells me that is all I'm allowed to say about our courtship story!

***Ann:*** Shortly after that, Joan and Duncan moved into my little house. Joan spent the first two years telling me it was just a temporary arrangement. But when we joined our money together, this was an important symbolic marker. Joan had been keeping books and kept insisting we contribute equally and telling me how much she owed me. I was making more money than she, and she was getting more and more into debt when I finally just said 'This is ridiculous'. So we pooled our money. I think one of the major issues in relationships is how money gets handled. When people keep their money separate, it's often a powerful metaphor around commitment.

Over the years we have faced many situations in which we have come out in different contexts. It is interesting to me that the coming out process is something that goes on over 50 years, hour by hour and day by day.

***Joan:*** One of the major decisions about coming out happened in the early 1990s when I was asked to give a plenary on gay and lesbian families at the

American Family Therapy Academy annual conference. Soon after that, I was asked to write a chapter on the same theme. These events required a kind of re-evaluation of my professional life. I had the idea that if I came out professionally I would be discredited as a family therapist in my town, I would be given a single kind of identity and status in the world – as a professional lesbian – and this frightened me. But the more I began to think and study and practice in this area, the more fascinated I became. It was almost like becoming an anthropologist visiting my own people, a people that I hadn't known very well or understood. I found it incredibly exciting, and have been working in that area ever since, for the last ten years.

Coming out to family is often the most complex of processes, and it too continues over the years. When Ann and I were celebrating our 25 years together I called up my mother to let her know. I said to her, 'We're having a big party next week to celebrate out 25th anniversary'. This was greeted with absolute silence. I really thought this was her chance, that she could send a card, or just offer some acknowledgment, so I went on. I said, 'We're having 25 to 30 people over to try to celebrate our time together'. Again there was silence. After the party I rang her up again, described the wonderful party we had had, and I said, 'Ann gave me a most beautiful diamond ring'. Again there was silence, and then she finally blurted out, 'Don't you have enough jewellery?' It was clear that after 25 years we still had a long way to go! And we continue to work on it.

***Ann:*** But the event that did make a difference, for Joan's mother, my family, many of our straight friends, and for Joan and me was Duncan and Meg's wedding. Weddings, of course, are powerful rituals, and all sorts of family issues arise in their planning and during the event itself. When Duncan and Meg decided to get married, the young couple had to inform Meg's family that Duncan was not Jewish, and then that they were lesbian. Meg's mother was deceased and her father, who was in his seventies, said, 'That's nice, dear'. He'd never met one, but he was willing to go with the flow. Then came more complex issues such as 'How do you define who your parents are?' Duncan's father was still living at the time but it had been Joan and I who had primarily raised him. Who was to be acknowledged? Meg's father had just re-married, and Meg had only known her step-mother a short time. These

I think were the hardest issues of all, how to work out whom you going to publicly acknowledge as family.

Meg and Duncan were very thoughtful about it all. They invited us out to dinner, and asked us what we thought they ought to put on the invitations. We wouldn't tell them what we thought they ought to do, but they wanted to know how Joan and I felt about both being on the invitation. And we were able to say very clearly that we wanted to be there as Duncan's family. We were throwing the party, after all, we were sharing the costs with Meg's family, and many of our friends would be coming to the wedding. But more than that, it was a public claiming, especially for me, the other mother.

***Joan:*** I was able to tell them that I thought it was very important that Ann be acknowledged on the wedding invitation after a lifetime of supporting Duncan and raising him. Throughout Duncan's childhood, Duncan adored Ann. She was a wonderful, loving positive parent. She was also very strong about Duncan maintaining a relationship with his father. Ann had lost her own father through a divorce when she was 18 months old and was determined that Duncan not experience a similar loss. In fact, she felt so strongly that one of our major arguments in those years was my wanting more protection from Duncan's father, who intruded on our lives, didn't respect the limits and boundaries that had been legally established, and wasn't meeting his responsibilities. But Ann was determined that we make it possible for Duncan's relationship with him to be supported. At times, it meant shoring him up. At the same time, although Ann was Duncan's primary parent in so many ways, it was very difficult for her to feel personally legitimate as a parent.

***Ann:*** Growing up in a culture that sees you as illegitimate has its hurtful effects, but we have enjoyed a most extraordinarily loving and positive family. About eight years ago Duncan came to me and told me 'You can call me your son'. In many ways it is the children who take the lead and who claim their family. Now the grandchildren are doing it too when they say to me, 'I just love you, Grandma', and I am learning to say 'My grandchildren'.

The day of Duncan and Meg's wedding was quite extraordinary. Walking down the aisle with Joan with Duncan between us was wonderful. We've always said that that day was our wedding too. It was the most beautiful definitional ceremony. There we were as Duncan's parents walking him down the aisle in front of everybody we knew – our family, my family, Joan's family, Meg's family and friends from everywhere. There was a whole community to witness this event and everybody was in tears. It was a public recognition of all of our relationships. It was Duncan and Meg's wedding, and as it turned out, it was also a ceremony for the two of us.

***Joan:*** For the first 25 years of our relationship, I would say to myself, 'I'm not lesbian, it's just that I love Ann. If something were to happen to Ann I'd probably get married again, or be in a relationship with a man.' I'm not so sure about this now. I feel very strongly committed as a lesbian, and that word for me symbolises a whole array of choices in relation to love, sex, and social and political commitments. It doesn't feel to me that I was a 'closet lesbian' who got in touch with her true self. That's never been the way I've put the story together. I think I keep becoming a lesbian. Even at 66 I'm still becoming a lesbian. And what that means to me changes from month to month and year to year.

***Ann:*** Perhaps I will end where I began this morning. In so many ways it is a new world for gay and lesbian people in the United States. We now live in an area of Massachusetts that is known as 'the happy valley' because it is a happy place for lesbians and gays, and there are many of us around. The irony is we didn't know this when we moved in. I went to school in the same area in the 1950s when it was a depressed mill town that had lost its mills. Now it's an up-scale rather sophisticated community with a visible population of gays and lesbians. We had no idea about this when we moved but it gradually dawned on us as we started meeting so many women couples and saw so many women holding hands in town. It's a new world. I say that a hundred times a week. I know we have a long way to go. I know young people are impatient, and I don't blame them, but if you had told me when I was thirty years old what the world would look like today in the States in relation to lesbian and gay rights, I would not have believed you.

***Joan:*** In contrast to the decades of silence, we'd like to tell you three brief stories involving our grandchildren that I think are about speaking the unsaid in such wonderfully positive and validating ways.

The first story occurred three years ago when Hannah was three, she came home with an album from school called 'A Family Is ...' Each page consisted of a photograph or two and a statement from the child about what a family meant to him or her. I think it was about page five before we got to a two parent nuclear heterosexual family, that disappearing family that every other family is compared to negatively.

The second story occurred in Julian's toddler room this year, the school sent a letter to all families explaining that one of the young teachers, a female named Hope, was transitioning to a social male named Jake over the holidays. The school then held a meeting for parents with experts on 'trans' present. It was the most positive kind of meeting, most parents concerned mainly about how to answer their children's questions in a good way and how this might challenge their ideas about gender.

***Ann:*** And the third little story is that our darling 5 year old Hannah recently said to me, 'You know, Baboo, you and Grandma could go someplace and get married and then come back here and you would be married'. (The state of Vermont, just north of us has established legal civil unions for same sex partners.)

These are wonderful silence breaking stories in our current lives.

# 2

# Anti-nuclear family practices

by

Claire Ralfs

The background to this paper is that my political consciousness was born in the anti-uranium movements of the late '70s and early '80s in South Australia. I also wish to acknowledge that in speaking on Kaurna land[2] – my hometown – that this land has shaped and inspired me in so many ways – some of which I wish to share with you today.

Family is complex. I have spent many years in discussion and reflection with my family about ways to describe and live family. It has been my partner Suzy and her love of words that has consistently stated that family is a verb – a doing word – a series of actions. Doing family is one of my daily challenges as it is for many of us. The chores and responsibilities never cease yet my family provides me with inspiration and courage and love and direction.

All of this sounds strikingly like right wing family values rhetoric! Because I passionately believe in the central role of my family and because this sounds like the conservative family mantra, I have had to get clearer about the difference between my version and theirs.

Suzy's reminder that family is a verb has been helpful to me in realising that it is not just *who* is in my family but rather the *practices of family* that change the concept. In reflecting and discussing this, we have come to name these practices *anti-nuclear family practices*.

Anti-nuclear family is not about the type of individuals in the family, but is about actively bringing people together with each other, across culture, across generation, across sexuality and into connection with the environment. In my experience, anti-nuclear family is about connection rather than atomising, collectivity rather than individualism. It is an eco-system of energy, loving and resources that circulate.

The nuclear family does not represent many people's lived experience of family. However the nuclear family construct is the template from which our welfare systems, our popular culture, our economic arrangements and education systems operate. The mum, dad and kids is what is meant when family is said. Ultimately it has been my experience that children are profoundly impacted by this and every child within my family has tried at times to fit our family into the nuclear family template. While this has not always been easy, it has made for very interesting conversations with our children about family.

Last week my 8 year old niece brought home her first homework sheet. She brought it next door to me – as one of her homework aunties – to help her complete it the night before it was due. One of the tasks was for her to name her family and their favourite foods. Now this child does not live with a nuclear family however she had her mother, father and biological sister all drawn in and favourite foods identified. When I asked her what about the rest of us she said – "no they only want to know about mum, dad and sister". We discussed this and she was very pragmatic and declared that she was in a hurry and was only going to give them what they wanted.

In claiming family as action I do not wish to ignore the powerful ties of biology. However I do believe that biology has been the privileged framework for recognising connections between people. I am still trying to fathom the role of biology and particularly its entitlements and impact on relationships.

When I was 18 years old I gave a child up for adoption. That child is now 22 years old and over the past 9 months I have had contact with him. The hazards for connections between relinquishing mothers and children grown into adults are many. Not least of these hazards is the poverty of relationship options available within the dominant nuclear family template and heterosexual dominance. At what point do you tell your adult son you've never met that you're a lesbian?

My son has a birth mother and a mother who parented him. I only held him for five minutes, and while I can still see his baby face I never heard him cry and I never watched him learn or grow.

He has a mother who did all these things and loves him and shared his growing and guided him in his childhood and now adulthood. So my son has a mother and birth mother. Culturally this is difficult. The invitations for birth mothers and mothers of adopted children to compete or not get on or be uncomfortable with each other are numerous. Unlike the many indigenous communities I know and love, in the non-indigenous community, multiple mothers is a problem rather than an advantage.

In reconnecting with my son I want to take the lead from my indigenous mentors and make multiple mothers a blessing. I want to challenge the dominant nuclear family that limits the ways we can describe our family connections.

In my loving of my sister Lynette, who grew up in an orphanage and my chosen daughter Roxanne who only joined the family 12 months ago at the age of 21 years old, there is a constant requirement to explain who is 'really' my sister or daughter. Biologically nuclear family connections are what is meant by real.

Recently, when Amy met my son – her brother - he introduced her as his 'half sister' – a biological description. Roxanne who was also there asked what was meant by half sister? After reflection, Amy and her new brother decided to drop the half bit.

Naming family connections is so important – being allowed to claim family is part of how we create belonging and honour loving. The nuclear family template is a shallow and I believe toxic framework in which our complex connections are divided and limited.

Naming anti-nuclear family practices is an invitation for us all to decommission the nuclear family – to take a stand against the dividing practices of the nuclear family. Anti-nuclear practices are an encouragement to focus on our meaningful connections with loved ones. If we can learn to do this in our daily life with our most intimate relationships perhaps we can also learn to be a family of humans who together may decommission the nuclear age.

## Note

1. The Kaurna people are the traditional custodians of the land on which the city of Adelaide now stands. In Australia, it is becoming customary, as a sign of respect, to acknowledge the Indigenous Australian peoples of the land prior to speaking at a formal event like a conference.

# 3

# Family as a verb

by

Suzy Stiles

It's quite extraordinary to be standing up here with some of my family – with my partner Claire, with Amy and with David – as well as with these other representatives of wonderful and proud families of difference.

It has been a long journey getting to this point. Being able to get up in front of you all and say 'hey, I'm part of a family worth talking about' or even 'Hey, I'm part of this family' hasn't come easy.

Sometimes those of us who are making family in unusual ways have trouble seeing ourselves as family, let alone making sure we are visible to other people. As a woman who has never given birth, I enjoy various parenting, auntying and other relationships to the many children in my life. So this forum is a great gift to our visibility, and I thank you all for it.

Part of the journey of getting here has been the process of creating a vision of ourselves as family, when for me what we are and what we do looks nothing like the middle-class family I grew up in the South of England (mum, dad and two kids). This was the regular model, and alternatives were few and far between. I certainly didn't know any families with two mums in them. Despite the strong, loving relationships in my family of origin, the nuclear family template has been a powerful constraining force, and getting to the point of being part of making and celebrating my family of difference has been an evolving process.

There were other complexities for me in thinking about standing up here to talk about my experience of family. As in many families there are rawnesses. Things aching to be completed. Hidden and difficult and scary things. Was I going to have to deny these, and stand up and be part of an advertisement for anti-nuclear families? Would it be safe to admit that not all is rosy and perfect in our struggles to make family together?

Thankfully I had a good talk to David, who reminded me that many people here could well share a sense of such complexities. Perhaps it would open up opportunities for these complexities to be spoken. I started to get very excited at the possibilities. So, having shared my fears, I'd like to share my hopes.

One strong hope I have is that by talking about our anti-nuclear family practices, maybe we can help expand the visions of what is possible in making family. Maybe more of us can see ourselves as belonging to 'families of difference', and celebrate the different ways we go about making family, however our families may be configured or named according to birth or marriage or relationships of choice.

My image of nuclear family is somehow inextricably linked to 'What is an Atom?' – an educational film which I saw as a child at school. Protons, neutrons and electrons were solid little billiard balls attracting, repelling and bouncing predictably around the screen in the darkened classroom.

The identity of an atom turned out to be far more complex – all those quarks, positrons and alpha beta particles. The family turned out to be far more complex too. Few people I know would describe their family as a nuclear family. The Australian census bears out this experience – only a small minority here live in a social unit which we would recognise as a nuclear family. But somehow the nuclear family lives on in the discourse of family in the West, despite the majority of so-called 'blended' families, single mums, single dads, the extended families of many different cultures, adoption, fostering and gay and lesbian relationships.

Like Claire, my understanding of family is shaped by my political experience. As a lesbian feminist and an anti-nuclear campaigner in London in the '80s, I objected to nuclear bombs, nuclear waste – and nuclear families. To my mind, both The Bomb and The Family had a lot to answer for. At the time I also fell in love with Community, which seemed a much nobler place than family, and I became a community artist.

Since then I have done a bit more thinking about the complexities of family, and also have been actively engaged in making one. I came to Australia in the late '80s, and have been privileged to meet and learn from many indigenous people here. Through their generous sharing I have seen that family has the capacity to be a very different thing – aunties can mother, and have more than the rather distant role I knew from my own childhood.

Making family and making community are no longer for me separable ideas, or acts. Children are part of a community, as much as they are part of family. As Ngarrindgeri cultural worker, community builder and good friend Major Sumner said to me one day, 'It takes a whole street to bring up a child, whether that street knows it or not'.

The making of family is a practice, and we have choices in this making. Which is why I encourage you to start using family as a verb, not a noun. An act of doing and being, not a descriptive category. A way of creating and sustaining relationships of support, caring, challenge and provocation.

I'd like to tell a story which celebrates the power of children as active makers of family. In particular to remember how Amy was the person who first invited me into making family.

It was about twelve years ago. Amy was seven. And I have to say, not wild about the fact that I was in a new relationship with her mother. Despite this, she must have had a good eye for my 'familying' potential, and given her fairly recent experience of the breakdown of Claire's previous relationship, decided she had better take things in hand. She asked me to write a letter to her in which I promised faithfully to be her auntie, and to keep on being her auntie, whatever happened. She insisted that I sign and date it properly and I had to keep it at all times in my wallet. She regularly used to open up my wallet and check that I still had it there. Sadly this wallet was stolen a few years later, or I would be able to produce it now as documentary evidence.

I love that Amy did this. It was such a powerful invitation to family, and she and I have gone on in our leaping ups and bumpy downs in familying together since. Being named and naming myself as auntie gave a framework for our connection. It also gave our relationship some authority and legitimacy to the world. Amy could introduce me to her friends and they immediately felt they understood our relationship. It needed no further justification, and I could safely appear in her stories about her life.

The naming as auntie also brought complexities. On her eighth birthday, Amy had a pyjama party for several of her school friends. Having introduced me as 'auntie' to her friends, it was not going to work if at the end of the evening I proceeded to go to bed with her mother. The naming that had enabled us to make family was invisibilising my relationship with Claire.

This naming also made it very clear that I was not a parent. Given the powerful framework of heterosexual dominance that Amy had to deal with at school, there was no way I was going to get invited to Parent/Teacher meetings. Working out my role in this was hard and at times I felt excluded, angry at the homophobic world and how we had all been limited by it.

As Amy has grown, and as we all have grown, we have struggled together to find other namings and other ways of being that support and make visible our relationships in familying together. For a while Amy and I settled for 'my partner's daughter' and 'my mother's partner' when describing each other, but this wouldn't do either. Where was our relationship with each other in this description? We haven't yet found a name which honours both the relationship between me and Amy and between me and Claire. It's lucky we know that familying is a verb, because we are still working on it.

I am now firmly and actively auntie to several other most extraordinary children, through choice, through my relationship with Claire and through my biological sister Jenny, who moved here from England, so inviting was our 'family of difference'.

Poppy and Essie are next door. Ella and Robin – six houses up the road. Sophie and Annie – a five minute walk away. All of them live within a square mile of us. For them we can be Homework Aunties, Lolly Aunties, the Salad Police, regular Monday or Wednesday night aunties, and of course, the Lecture Aunties, always to be relied upon to provide challenging opinions.

Becoming an auntie can happen at any time I have discovered. A delight of the past year has been that Roxanne, as a young woman of 21, has been choosing to make family with Claire, Amy and myself.

Finally I'd like to touch on another long journey in familying which I have been part of for many years now. Claire and I wanted to have a baby together. We wanted to do so with a father who would make a relationship with this child. We believed that our extended and wonderful family was a great place for another baby to start the journey of familying.

I won't take you to all the highways and byways that this road took us. A lot is too raw to talk about right now. Our journey drew to a close with a miscarriage last year. David has been our great friend through this, would-be father and fellow traveller on our long journey. Although we did not have a baby together, we have made family and continue to do so.

David has written a beautiful song which he would like to sing about this. So I'll stop talking and let him sing.

# 4

# Eulogy

by

David Denborough

This eulogy was originally written and sung for purely personal reasons but sharing it here with a wider audience is for broader purposes. I hope that perhaps it can offer company to those who have had losses that are difficult to put into words or share with others. Many people who live outside of the mainstream for whatever reason experience losses that are not easy to speak about or to share. Finding ways to create alternative rituals, poems and songs to name such experiences seems worthwhile.

I believe it is a significant loss (both for individuals and the culture more broadly) that child rearing is generally accepted only within heterosexual paradigms. In saying this however, I am conscious that there are many other emotions and meanings associated with living life without children, both in my own life and more generally. For many people, not to be involved in bringing a child into the world is a personal and political choice. For me, I have known since the age of twelve that I would never want to raise a child within a nuclear family structure. For many others, with life involving so many different challenges, delights and explorations child-raising is simply not a priority.

Having said all of this, I do believe it is a loss for this culture that child-rearing remains relatively unavailable to those living outside conventional heterosexual relationships. This sung eulogy is my personal way of acknowledging this loss. It is dedicated to all of us who have had losses that are hard to explain.

It is a little difficult to express on paper what was written as a song, but I hope some of the spirit of the melody is conveyed here …

*How do you say farewell*
*to someone*
*whom you've never met*
*and will never see?*
*Do you compose a eulogy*
*To sing to the moon,*
*the stars*
*and the sea?*

*Or do you gather*
*with new family,*
*made from*
*sharing turkey-basters*
*and sweet sweet dreams?*
*Do you re-tell the stories*
*of pregnancy lost*
*and friendships found?*

*As you celebrate*
*the births around you*
*do you glance away*
*discretely?*
*As you watch your parents*
*growing older*
*do you marvel at all*
*of life's mysteries?*

*Do you find yourself*
*asking questions*
*Of your own birth,*
*mothers, daughters and sons?*
*Do you feel somehow older,*
*both sad and*
*so grateful at life*
*all in one?*

*How can I convey*
*to my new family*
*what it meant to*
*spend those nights together?*
*All the humour,*
*gentleness and dignity,*
*trying to create new life,*
*we gave it our best show...*

*How do you say farewell to someone*
*whom you've never met*
*and will never see?*
*Do you compose a eulogy*
*To sing to the moon,*
*the stars*
*and the sea...?*
*I guess we'll see*

# 5

# Amy's story

*This paper was written in 1995 when Amy was a 13 year old high school student who chose to be known only by her first name in this context.*

Difference is found everywhere: in homes, in shops, in workplaces, in schools. Difference is a fact of life, and the more it is openly identified and discussed the more it can be understood.

In schools, being noticeably different can be horrible. You can be teased mercilessly by other children, and sometimes the teachers don't even do anything about it, mostly probably because they are of the same opinion.

What if you or your family are different, but in a way which isn't immediately noticeable? How do you cope with degrading remarks about your lifestyle? Comments which aren't directed at you, but nonetheless are about you can be very painful. Do you listen to them and laugh with their jokes and pretend that it doesn't concern you, like I have done? Or do you make a stand against their unfair remarks, as I can do now?

You see, my mother is a lesbian, and although I don't think there is anything wrong with that, a lot of people in my life seem to have thought that. And, believe me, sitting around listening to your best friends humiliating your life is not much fun. School is the place where such humiliation often occurs for children. I know that, for me, school was often a place where I was exposed to much misunderstanding of my family's lifestyle.

When I was younger; it took great difficulty and a lot of planning for me to have a friend sleep over. I was very careful about who I let know my mum was a lesbian. If I was to tell a friend about my mother, it was after a lot of careful watching and anticipation to see what their reaction would be. I would be on my guard all the time to detect the slightest bit of bias against lesbians or homosexuals. In fact, the first time I told anyone I was about 7 years old. I wrote on a slip of paper, 'My Mum is a lesbian', and gave it to my friend. All the careful watching and decision-making paid off when she turned around and gave me a big hug,

I wasn't so lucky the next time. I told another friend, and it was OK for a while, and then when she and I had an argument, she told the whole class. It was awful: I got teased and stirred all day. My mother had to go to the school and complain to the principal. I was so scared that it would make it worse, but my mother insisted that it shouldn't be happening. The principal didn't really do anything, but he was very polite to me and eventually the teasing stopped.

After this, I was very scared to be different. Although I was friends with the Aboriginal and Khmer kids in my class, I wasn't best friends with them because I didn't want to stand out. I often hated the way the Aboriginal kids were talked about, but I felt unable to do much about it. Towards the end of my primary schooling, there was a lovely Maori girl who came to our class. She was treated really badly. I was friends with her and tried to protect her, but I was still scared to be too outspoken about it. She really showed me how to stand up to the teasing. I didn't get to know her as well as I would have liked, because she decided to leave the school shortly after arriving. I eventually followed her example and went to another school to get away from the horrible attitudes and pressure to conform.

Now every time I think about the way I and anybody who had different ideas was treated, I feel really angry and bitter. All the effort that I put into trying to be friends with those girls was just wasted time.

Now I can see that, at my primary school, it was assumed that we would be what was accepted as normal, heterosexual. So if anyone talked about the possibility of being homosexual, or teased someone about being a 'poofter' or a 'leso', the teachers would often pass it off as childish pranks. There was never any attempt by the teachers to make different family backgrounds understood or acceptable. In this environment, the prejudiced ideas of my circle of 'friends' were left to flourish, hurting people, including me, in its path.

Now I am at a girls' high school and it is a very different situation to the one I had been used to. In the second term of being at this school, we had long discussions over several weeks about the reality of being homosexual, and through this I had the opportunity to hear other people's opinions about the subject. When the discussions first started, I felt quite scared that I was about to be exposed. As the discussions continued though, I became more comfortable because I started to see that not everyone was against homosexuality. This was a great relief.

The teachers at my high school are more open to all sorts of difference. Different religions and cultures are acknowledged and actively respected. The teachers also talk about different types of families, so a family isn't just presented as two kids and a mother and a father. I have quickly come to develop quite a high level of respect for my teachers due to this aspect of their teaching. And while there is still the idea of normality, it is not just expected.

This has had a really big impact on my daily life. When I was with friends from primary school, I was very guarded and unrelaxed, always expecting to be cut down. In the friendships I have been able to form at my present school, I have come to appreciate laughter and the feeling of being accepted.

When I think about my primary school friends, I feel angry about how they treated me, but I also feel sort of sorry for them. Their prejudice really narrows what they are able to experience. I believe that the way the teachers at my present school have made it possible for the students from different lifestyles or cultural and religious backgrounds to be valued members of the school community is crucial to the quality of my education. It's not just the children from 'different' backgrounds that this benefits. Everyone benefits, including children from 'normal' families because they get to learn about the world around them.

The longer I am at this school, I am getting more confident about standing up for myself, and others. I know now that everyone is an individual, and that's about as normal as it gets.

# 6

# Amy Ralfs' story

*This paper was written in 1999 when Amy Ralfs was 17.*

In 1995 I wrote a story. It was Amy's story and it told of my life as the daughter of a lesbian and how this affected my experiences of education. Since that time, the response I have received from those who read my article has helped give me the strength to change my story. For a lot of my life I felt that my lifestyle was too different to talk about. I felt vulnerable around most other young people and was convinced that my sort of lifestyle did not exist outside my family and most definitely not at my primary school! Since the publication of my article, in which I was identified only by my first name, I have received some inspiring feedback, in particular that from other young people. This feedback told me that what I had written had helped them fight feelings of 'abnormality' and this has been very powerful for me. This to me shows the importance of young people having peers from a diverse range of backgrounds. This, in my opinion, can help them to be themselves and to value who they are.

When I wrote my story, it was only as Amy. At that point I would not have been able to identify myself without the fear of recognition. This fear stemmed from a belief that recognition of my situation would ultimately lead to rejection. But today, I am here not only as Amy, but as Amy Ralfs, because now I can reveal who I am without that fear. In fact I was even able to invite my school principal to hear me speak today! My ability to do this is partly due to my recognition that my mother's lesbianism is only one of the many differences which help to make my life unique. The more I recognise the positive influences that these differences have on me, the more I am able to do away with many of my feelings of isolation and 'abnormality' which came from keeping such a big part of my life secret.

There are many people and aspects of my life which differ from the norm. My family is not merely those whom I am related to by blood, nor is it restricted to mother, father and siblings. I have many women in my life who have been signed up as 'aunties'; I have cousins who have been more like sisters; I have my mother's partner of ten years who has been like a parent to me in that time; I have an uncle who has been like a father (and is the most qualified unemployed person I have ever met!) and I can count people from various backgrounds among family and friends. While I find I have gained from living with and around so many different people, there seems an inability by others to accept them as my family. On my thirteenth birthday, when I introduced three women as aunts, my friends needed to sit down and try to work out the biological connections, rather than accept that they were people I considered family. I believe that it is necessary for the definition of family to be broadened and the conventional labels, which are all too readily employed, removed. In the eyes of present day society I would be viewed as the only child from a single parent family. However, to describe myself as this is to make invisible many of the people who play a part in my life. It has been this experience which has taught me to look for the stories behind the imposed labels. At one point these labels greatly affected my experience of the world outside my family, but now I have been able to see through their power. The restrictions inflicted by these classifications leave no room for your story to be heard, and this silencing can be very damaging.

The diverse array of people within my life has allowed me to challenge the concept of normality, which plagues so many young people in particular. In the face of what is portrayed as 'normal' in regards to family or lifestyle, it is often easy for young people to feel isolated and marginalised because they perceive themselves and their experiences to be 'abnormal'. From this position many come to disregard the invaluable learning that these experiences can provide. In my life, it is the incredible uniqueness of all of my family and friends and their acceptance of each other that allows me to be the individual that I am. The wide range of opinions gives me the opportunity to challenge and be challenged as well as discuss issues, and the many different life experiences help me to increase my understanding of the world.

However, while I have become much more at ease with my life and the people in it, I still at times find it necessary to explain myself to others. Recently, I was in this situation and had to tell a friend of my mother's lesbianism. It was not that previously I had been hiding it, but that it feels so normal to me that I forgot that it was something that was necessary to spell out. Her response when I told her was to me a very telling remark. She said: 'I thought so, but it's not exactly something you ask is it?' and she was right. Society is so geared towards heterosexuality being the accepted lifestyle that again this concept of 'normality' restricts us to blatantly accepting that that's what everyone will be. So far none of my friends have taken me aside to whisper in my ear: 'Amy – my mum's heterosexual'. Maybe if society wasn't so quick to label you as being one thing or another, it would not be necessary for whispering of this kind to take place. I believe that the more we can come to identify and value the positive influences that the different aspects of our lives have on us, the more genuinely we can know each other. The sooner we are able to stop using labels to classify people, the sooner we will be allowing ourselves the opportunity to enrich our own existences with a greater understanding of the stories of others. By living with the differences that exist in my life, I get a taste of the extent of diversity in the world. I am grateful for this opportunity because it means I know the value of listening to the marginalised voices of society.

# 7

# The love we leave behind us when we're gone

by

Christopher Behan & James Light

**Chris:** To begin to convey a little of what it means to live in our family, we'd like first to sing you a song. It is the lullaby we wish we were sung when we were children, and it is the lullaby we sing to our daughter, Eva. It's a song called 'Everything Possible' by Fred Small.

*We have cleared off the table,*
*the leftovers saved,*
*washed the dishes and put them away.*
*I have told you a story*
*and tucked you in tight*
*at the end of your knockabout day.*

*As the moon sets its sail to carry you to sleep*
*over the midnight sea*

*Well, I will sing you a song no one sang to me.*
*May it keep you good company.*

*You can be anybody that you want to be.*
*You can love whomever you will.*
*You can travel any country where your heart leads*
*and know I will love you still.*
*You can live by yourself.*
*You can gather friends around.*
*You can choose one special one.*
*And the only measure of your words and your deeds*
*will be the love you leave behind when you're gone.*

***Chris:*** Within my family, it is tradition for the bride or the groom to sing a song during wedding celebrations. When I first heard this song performed by a gay acapella choir called The Flirtations, I was so moved by the words, the melody and the group's perfect harmonies that I decided this was the song I wanted to sing when James and I held our commitment ceremony. This commitment ceremony had a lot to do with us becoming parents. We knew that we were soon to adopt a child from a woman called Cindy who was pregnant at that time. We didn't know exactly who was coming to live with us, we didn't know her name would be Eva, but we felt it was important that this baby would be born into a family where the partners had made some clear commitments to one another and had invited friends and family to witness them. We decided to hold a commitment ceremony and during it I sang.

I was standing in front of a room filled with a huge family and many friends. When I came to sing the line 'no one sang this song to me' I was looking directly at my father and he had tears in his eyes. I wasn't looking in an accusatory way. Back in the early 1960s, when I was being sung lullabies, this song literally didn't exist to sing. If it had, I think my dad probably would have sung it to me. He tried to support the kid that I was to the best of his ability, but all through my younger years I didn't know that it was possible to openly love another boy or man. I didn't know there was ever going to be a possibility that I could have a committed relationship with a man, or if I was going to be gay that I could ever have children. These didn't seem to be possibilities in that time and place. And so, when I sang this song at our commitment ceremony and saw my father crying in the audience, his tears meant the world to me.

My father died just after Eva was born and so I became a father just as I lost my own. Whenever I sing this song I think of him. It's not a sad song, it's beautiful, but it has bittersweet parts. It has since become a lullaby in our family. When Eva was a baby, and needed to be rocked to sleep, I rediscovered the song's beauty. Each time it is sung it reconnects me to our commitment ceremony, all those who witnessed it, and all those who are joined with us in raising our child.

***James:*** I come from a very small family in a very small fishing village of five hundred people. My parents owned the local diner. As far as anyone there is concerned, life for a man consists of getting married at 18 to someone who lives nearby, having children, and working for your parents until they retire and you take over their business. By the time I was twenty it was expected I would have a spouse and two children, a house with a white picket fence, a dog and a nice neighbourhood. In hindsight, all of this has come true, but it looks a little different than anyone back home would have predicted.

My mother refused to talk about the fact that I was gay. In fact the closest we ever came to a conversation about it was when she said one day: 'You know you're different than everybody else, so whatever you do, you should probably go away and do it somewhere else'. Before Chris and I had our commitment ceremony, Chris said to me, 'You have to find a way of having me acknowledged in a more open way. Otherwise, who will I ever be to your family?' And so we went to my parents' house. Chris and my father sat in the chair after dinner and watched TV while I took my mother for a walk. As we were walking I said to her, 'You know Ma we have to have a conversation about what's going on in my life, because I want to include you, I want to tell you about it.' At that precise moment my mother looked up at the sky, grabbed the back of her sweater, pulled it over her head and said 'It's starting to rain – RUN!' And she ran diagonally through a puckerbrush field, a field full of thistles, to get home. I realised then that there weren't going to be many conversations about my sexuality with my mother.

Recently though, after an equal rights vote was defeated in our state, my mother raised the topic with me. She said that she was surprised that the 'Gay Rights Bill' had been defeated. She said that everyone whom she had spoken with thought it would pass. She let me know that she had voted for the bill, that she could now say the word gay out loud, and that she was surprised that the state had voted it down. For someone who ran through the puckerbrush, this was quite an achievement.

Now, my mother is a big part of Eva's life. As a matter of fact early on she kept telling us, in a kind of bewildered way, what great parents we were. When Eva was a baby, I think she couldn't believe how tender we were with her. In her experience I guess men have not been tender. Caring for a baby involves a lot of gentle loving. My mother loved watching us feeding Eva, dressing her and caring for her. I think it was a revelation to her that we could be so sweet.

***Chris:*** But we are getting ahead of ourselves. Let's go back a few steps. After applying to adopt a child and being appraised by the state as to whether or not we would provide a good home, we were matched with Cindy when she was five months pregnant with a child she was not in a position to raise. We initially connected with Cindy on the phone. We talked and talked until we all decided that it seemed a good match, and so we travelled down to New Jersey, about six hours away, to meet in person. Once there, we negotiated with Cindy what kind of relationship she wanted to have with us. We decided together that Cindy would have our phone numbers and could call us if she wanted to. She decided she would like to have regular pictures of the child and some degree of contact. We set up the terms, made a commitment to one another and vowed to see how it all went from there. At this point, it was four and a half months before the baby was due.

***James:*** In so many ways, over the next four and a half months we felt pregnant with anticipation. We were nervous and poured over books about what it was like to be pregnant at seven months, at eight months, at nine months, and what the baby was like as the pregnancy progressed.

At the same time, much to my surprise, we also became closer and closer to Cindy. At first, I'd thought that she was simply going to be the person who was to give birth to our daughter, our baby. But gradually I realised that we were becoming family especially when Cindy made it clear that she wanted us to be her coaches at the birth. We prepared in every way that we could. Every form was filled out, checked and re-checked. Every book was read and re-read. We spoke with everyone we could think of. Our bags were packed, money was put aside, and the car was always ready. The minute Cindy went into labour her sister called us. We grabbed our bags, jumped in the car and were there in time to witness Eva coming into the world. A few minutes after Eva was born, Cindy turned to us and said, 'I feel like we just had a baby' and I said 'I think we did'.

I got to hold Eva when she was only one minute old and as cute as a button. Cindy said 'who wants to hold this baby?', and I said 'I do'. I had always thought that I was going to want to avoid a relationship with Cindy after the birth because of my own jealousies, fears and inadequacies. But the complete opposite turned out to be true. I feel more comfortable knowing Cindy, knowing who she is, knowing that she's proud of her daughter, that she's proud of her decision and that she's pleased to have us in her family. She calls us regularly to see how Eva's doing, but also just to talk to us as family. She calls to tell us how she's doing. When Cindy does something that she's proud of, she calls us because she knows we will be proud of her too. I don't think that she's found many other places for that. We found ourselves becoming quite protective of Cindy. While she was in hospital I was like a mother bear! I became her advocate in the hospital because people weren't being considerate of her needs and wishes.

***Chris:*** One of the most bittersweet parts of the process happened when it was time to leave the hospital. It was only when it was time to go separate ways that we really got in touch with what a profound act it was for Cindy to pass Eva over to us. I remember the day so clearly. We were all getting ready to leave the hospital on the same morning. Cindy, James and I all dressed Eva in a little outfit that we had bought. I remember her white jumper and a little white hat with polka dots. Cindy was talking and cooing to the baby and getting ready to leave when she passed the baby over to James.

We'd offered to give Cindy a ride home, but she really wanted to take a taxi. After what seemed like a very long time, we put Cindy in the taxi as we tried to place Eva in the backseat of our car in a baby seat. This transaction was taking place in the parking lot. Because of legalities the hospital wouldn't let it take place inside. As soon as we got Cindy into the taxi we just broke down and sobbed.

We had thought a lot about leaving the hospital but we hadn't understood how hard it was going to be for us and for Cindy. There we were, the two of us crying our eyes out trying to figure out how to get the baby into the car seat that we'd never used before, as Cindy drove away in the taxicab. It was all at once, one of the sweetest and the saddest moments in my life. It was one of the saddest things I have ever witnessed and at the same time one of the greatest things I've ever felt. I wasn't prepared to feel Cindy's loss and my own joy at the same time. The juxtaposition of what Cindy was offering to us and what we were going away with was beautifully and painfully manifest. In that moment a gratitude to Cindy awakened within me that I can never hope to convey here. In some ways it had been present from the moment I met her, but as I saw the taxi driving away I became differently aware of the significance of all that she has given to our family.

***James:*** Chris and I then drove about a mile to a park that we had noticed the day before. It was a beautiful day and we walked into the park down by the pond and sat under this huge oak tree. We opened Eva's bundle of blankets, took all her clothes off and just sat and stared at her. For the first time we were really able to examine her toes and just drink her in, because I didn't feel that we could do this in front of Cindy. I hadn't wanted Cindy to see too much of my joy, but of course I hadn't wanted to seem aloof either. There in the park it felt like we finally got to enjoy that first meeting of baby and parent. We sat under the tree and we fed her and got to know her. We relaxed, got back in the car and drove home.

That was the beginning of being a family with two dads. All along the way we have had to make our family up – to work out what roles we are going to play and how. I feel very fortunate that we have been able to invent our family in this way rather than have roles preconceived and named for us in advance. We have literally been involved in choosing the parenting practices that we believe we each do the best and that we feel the best about doing. I had every intention from the beginning of being in the more traditional role – what people would call the 'mummy' role. I wanted this. I begged for it. In fact I insisted on it, I'd have it no other way. When we are on the road, I'll be the one to have a snack in my bag and a bottle in my back pocket. I have made my schedule fit Eva's to a greater degree than we have adjusted Chris' schedule. And I am starting to take more participation in Eva's education. I am class mummy this year. We are making it up as we go along and I feel we are doing well. Responding to other people's reactions however, has at times been challenging.

When Eva was very little, I'd have a two week old baby in a carrier in the shopping cart in the grocery store and women would come up to me for no reason and ask me, 'Do you need some help?' 'Can I help you out?' 'Where's that baby's mother?'. I guess they were trying to be helpful but it would happen so often, and they would assume I was so hopeless, that over time it made me feel quite angry. So much so that it got to the point that I would say that her mother was dead as this seemed to shut down the conversations the fastest. I soon realised however that this wasn't fair to Eva or Cindy. Then when Eva got a little older, women would come up to her and say 'Oh your mummy must be so lucky that you're out with your daddy grocery shopping. We don't get that in my house'. We would just nod.

People seem genuinely shocked by the idea that a man could be the primary carer for a child, that a man could be always responsible for every care giving moment of a child's life. It is still assumed that men are kind of spare-part parents, or back-up parents. This assumption has meant that people have consistently come up to me and offered unsolicited advice about baby care. I'd be walking down the street with Eva and if she was crying people would just come up to me and start giving me advice about how to hold her, or how to burp her. It was very undermining.

This doesn't happen any more but now we are faced with different dilemmas. Up until recently, for example, it has been fine for me to accompany Eva when she goes into public toilets. Now as she gets older, however, that is becoming less acceptable. It can be scary for Eva and for us to send her alone into a highway restaurant's bathroom where there might be twenty-five people in the room. If Eva's nervous, I generally still accompany her. She's our daughter and her comfort and safety has to be our priority.

***Chris:*** I am very conscious that it's not just the two of us who are raising Eva. We are part of a larger community. When people are concerned about who Eva's female role models might be, there is so much I want to say to them. I want to say that I have never been interested in having the kind of a family in which one person is modelling the way to be a man while another is modelling the way to be a woman. I want to say that as a young man I had plenty of male role models but there weren't very many gay people who were living openly whom I could look at and say 'I want to be like them'. I want to say that people still don't seem determined that boys have access to older gay men as role models of ways of being male. I want to say that there are so many different ways to be in this world and perhaps that is what is most important to model. And I want to say that Eva is being raised by us and by a community of people within which our women friends, relatives and neighbours play enriching parts. Just as they are involved in helping us take care of Eva, we are involved in caring for their children.

***James:*** I'd like just to mention the woman after whom Eva is named. My great grandmother's name was Eva. Out of all the people I knew when I was growing up, my great grandmother and I were birds of the same feather even though she was in her nineties when I was around ten. I think she knew I was gay from the very beginning, although she would never have said that, even if she was alive today. Not only did I reach out to spend time with her but my family sent me to live with her each year from January until March. I was there to take care of her but I am not sure who was caring for who. With Granny Eva I would knit, cook and sew. I would show an interest and she would teach me. I remember going into the cellar and unearthing her old sewing machine. The first thing we made together was an apron out of yellow calico. When we would cook dinner together she couldn't lift the fry-pan and I couldn't reach the cupboards. She had been treated unkindly for much of her life and yet she was one of the most profoundly kind people I have ever met. She grew up in the nineteenth century and lived to be just over a hundred. She was my role model. When it came to naming our daughter, there was one name that stepped forward: Eva, after Granny Eva.

***Chris:*** To end our talk, I'd like to return to the words of our lullaby, especially the line: 'You can be anybody that you want to be'. I wanted to be a parent and I have become one, even though nobody gave me permission. Some people have said to me 'Aren't you just a parent because you were socially inculcated in a heterosexual culture to want to be a parent?' And I say maybe. All I know is that I spent a good part of my twenties grieving the fact that, because of my sexuality, I wasn't going to be a father. Maybe this grief was due to dominant cultural expectations, but in my late twenties I came to terms with the fact that I wasn't going to be a dad. I came to see being gay as a gift and recognised how it meant I could do lots of other things with my life. It was only in meeting James who was so sure that he wanted to be a father that I became convinced that it was a good idea.

And now I am singing lullabies to my daughter to make sure that she has permission to be anybody that she wants to be, to love anybody that she chooses. By singing these words, we are also anticipating the future. We are preparing ourselves to make space for Eva to be anybody who she wants to be. Maybe she'll end up being a Republican. Maybe she'll choose not to be a parent and so we will never be grandparents. We try hard to question some of the myths that shape the dreams of young girls. When Eva says 'when I grow up and get married and have children', we say 'well maybe you won't get married' or 'maybe your partner will be a girl' or 'maybe you won't have a partner'. In different ways, the song is preparing all of us for the future, preparing us to think through what kind of love we want to leave behind us when we're gone.

To complete this talk we'd now all like to sing this song one last time, and we invite you all to join us.

## *Everything Possible*

by

Fred Small

*We have cleared off the table, the leftovers saved,*
*Washed the dishes and put them away*
*I have told you a story and tucked you in tight*
*At the end of your knockabout day*
*As the moon sets its sails to carry you to sleep*
*Over the midnight sea*
*I will sing you a song no one sang to me*
*May it keep you good company.*

*CHORUS:*
*You can be anybody you want to be,*
*You can love whomever you will*
*You can travel any country where your heart leads*
*And know I will love you still*
*You can live by yourself, you can gather friends around,*
*You can choose one special one*
*And the only measure of your words and your deeds*
*Will be the love you leave behind when you're gone.*

*There are girls who grow up strong and bold*
*There are boys quiet and kind*
*Some race on ahead, some follow behind*
*Some go in their own way and time*

*Some women love women, some men love men*
*Some raise children, some never do*
*You can dream all the day never reaching the end*
*Of everything possible for you.*

*Don't be rattled by names, by taunts, by games*
*But seek out spirits true*
*If you give your friends the best part of yourself*
*They will give the same back to you.*

*CHORUS:*
*You can be anybody you want to be,*
*You can love whomever you will*
*You can travel any country where your heart leads*
*And know I will love you still*
*You can live by yourself, you can gather friends around,*
*You can choose one special one*
*And the only measure of your words and your deeds*
*Will be the love you leave behind when you're gone.*

Reprinted with permission. A live recording of this song by Fred Small can be found on 'Everything Possible' available from Flying Fish Records, 1304 West Schubert, Chicago, IL 60614 USA. For sheet music of this song and others by Fred Small go to Yellow Moon Press at www.yellowmoon.com

# 8

# Making ourselves up as we go along

by

*Jane Speedy*

I'd like to just tell you a few short stories about my family. The word family is one I have often felt a little confused about, as it refers to both my family of genetic origin and what I might describe as my 'family of choice' but also, perhaps to a more global sense of family and to many imaginings and hopes about being in a family.

In some ways the main reason that I ever got to come to Adelaide in the first place (which is about as far away from Bristol, England, as you can get) was because of a shared sense of family with some of the other people giving this keynote address, even though I had never met them.

My partner, Sarah and I were so overexcited to be pregnant and so proud of our baby daughter, Esther, that it took a while after she was born for us to remember that not everybody was going to be as thrilled with us and our family as we were. It was when we first hit the primary school system that we realised how much other people's ideas about lesbian families might have a major impact on Esther, and on the way she saw herself and us. It was around that time that a friend sent me a copy of 'Amy's story'.

This was a story that Amy Ralfs (who you have just heard from) wrote about her experiences in primary school. Some of those experiences were not so good and what she wrote about was quite hard to read, but what shone through were her courage and determination and her strong sense of family. I was very moved by Amy's writing and set out to find out more about the place that had published her story, which is how I found out about the Dulwich Centre and its work.

When my daughter Esther was about seven I gave her Amy's story to read, and although she has been brought up in a different part of the world, in a different time and her experience of primary school has been very different, she has always been really pleased to have Amy's story. Esther has always known other lesbian and gay families, and has read books written by grownups about these kinds of families in North America, but it was very different and very special to read something written by another child, in a lesbian family who was living in Australia, right across the other side of the world.

There are now four of us in our immediate family, my partner Sarah, myself, Esther, who is now 8and 3/4, and Shaena who is a golden retriever. One of the things we get regularly asked, or that gets regularly asked about us, is which one of us is the 'real' mum. This often feels like a pretty loaded question. It's something that lots of people seem to want to know and it's quite hard to answer. Is it the one of us who gave birth to Esther, in which case I am the real mum? Is it the one of us who has spent more time at home, doing the kind of things that mums do, and is currently at home looking after her daughter while I swan off to Australia to give a talk about our family, in which case, Sarah is 'real mum'?

I have often felt quite angry about this question, and have regularly been quite badly behaved in the sort of answers I have come up with…

But I have had a lot to learn from my own mum who has not always found it that easy to be pleased about some of my life choices. Just before she died she was asked, for the umpteenth time, which one of us was Esther's real mum, and her reply was:

> 'Well, I'm not sure that either of them is, actually … If you ask me, they're both just making it all up as they go along …'

And I have to say this was an absolutely brilliant answer in a number of ways, firstly because it completely floors and silences all comers. Secondly because it was a quiet and loving recognition on my mum's part that Sarah was a parent and a significant and important person in her granddaughter's life which is not something that my mum had found it easy to acknowledge, and also because it says something positive to the world about what it might be like being part of a family for whom there may not be so many predictions and expectations about how we are going to live our lives.

My guess is that most parents make most of it up as they go along for most of the time, but that somehow being a family a little outside the run-of-the-mill, we have had more permission to do that, and having us around may give other people greater permissions too. For instance, a year or so ago, Esther's class at school were treated to the standard BBC (British Broadcasting Corporation) TV program on how babies are made, and in the classroom discussion that followed, Esther, who is one of at least three children in her year at school who also have two mums, piped up with:

'Can I just say that that's not how we did it'?

She then proceeded to give a graphic and detailed description of our particular version of donor insemination, a process that took place with a friend of ours and how she now felt especially connected with him, his partner and his two daughters, her two half sisters, with whom she loves to spend time. According to Esther's teacher at the time, this was not the kind of discussion that had been anticipated, but that hearing Esther talk about one different way of making a baby opened up a discussion of several other children's versions of 'how they did it'. It transpired that in Esther's year at school there were families with IVF babies and adopted babies and fostered babies and a whole range of family set-ups and arrangements that had not, hitherto, really ever been talked about. Having one family that was quite explicitly making itself up as it went along and even taking some pride in this, had perhaps opened the lid on these conversations for other people as well.

One of the tricky bits about talking about my family in this kind of setting, knowing that these are stories that rarely get this kind of airtime, is that a large part of me wants to paint a really rosy picture of the ways that we live our lives, if only to counteract the many negative and prejudiced views of lesbian and gay lives and families that abound. To give a more honest account of my family, and myself however, I would have to say that it has not all been rosy and that, as with most people, our stories have been quite complicated and quite messy and some of our experiences as a family have been quite hard.

One of the most painful things that has happened to us was that a year after Esther was born Sarah and I found that we could not bear to carry on living together any longer. We both loved our young daughter dearly but didn't seem to be able to love or even like each other very much any more. This was a really hard thing to happen. There had been a lot of adverse publicity around that time about lesbian and gay parenting. The British 'child protection act' had been passed just before Esther was born which had included many important clauses to do with children's rights. It had also included the notorious clause 28 that described families like ours as 'pretended families' and had expressly prevented, by law, any 'promotion' of pretended families by government agencies.

We had been very involved at the time in protests against clause 28. We still are. We had argued that our families were just as real and loving and just as complex as many others and that the views expressed by certain members of the (then conservative) government that gays and lesbians were usually in unsuitable and unstable relationships that did not last were unjust views that came from positions of ignorance and prejudice.

And yet here we were, a little while later, splitting up as a couple. We were both captured by a sense of guilt, of letting the side down, of having betrayed Esther and the lesbian and gay people in our community. I remember telling a heterosexual colleague at work about the break-up, to which she replied 'ah, well, that often happens in those kinds of relationships'. A year or so earlier I might have given quite a lengthy and certainly a very noisy and robust response to this kind of remark At the time I just sat there in silence, constrained by misery and shame.

Looking back now on this period of our lives, which lasted about five years, it was a very painful time, but it is also the time in the history of our little family that I can look back on with the most pride.

One of the extraordinary, instant, and fairly universal responses to our change in living circumstances was that as soon as we moved into separate houses I was treated as a single parent and Sarah became 'invisible'. Sarah was legally a parent and morally a parent and in the day-to-day life of our family was very much an equal parent. Esther spent her time pretty equally between our two households and never thought of herself as having anything less than two mothers. Yet, somehow it was incredibly hard to get this acknowledged. Schools, grandparents, friends and other family members were all able to recognise that Sarah, now labelled my ex-partner, would have some involvement with 'my' child, but the idea that she might be equally involved or even sometimes more involved with Esther's parenting than I was, seemed to go against the grain.

We have thought a lot about why this might have been … after all, many families share their day-to-day lives between two homes and in living this lifestyle, Esther was no different from many other children in her class at school … In fact Esther is still connected to at least four households locally that she might call home, alongside a number of children in our neighbourhood, so what was the problem?

Perhaps it has something to do with the ways our culture uses the word lesbian and what might be a routinely thought of comfortable definitions of that word. It may suit people to think of this word as defining us in terms of our sexual relationships and activities. Breaking out of those definitions and describing ourselves also in terms of our parenting practices, our ways of creating and living in families, or our moral, ethical and spiritual commitments to each other, may not seem so comfortable.

Perhaps it has something to do with the 'throw away' culture of parenting and family lives that has gained a certain currency in Britain at the moment. It is not unusual for children to virtually lose all connection with one or other of their parents and it is pretty commonplace to have much less contact with a parent who moves out of the family home.

For whatever reasons, Sarah's unquestioning commitment to her daughter and my absolute trust and faith in her commitment to sharing parenting with me was somehow troubling, confusing and uncomfortable for quite a lot of people. It certainly 'troubled' and surprised our own expectations of our relationship.

Gradually through our conjoint efforts, Sarah has become a more and more visible parent. This has been an achievement that we all take a sense of pride in. Sarah's quiet persistence in developing an 'ethics of lesbian parenting' has been very moving and heart-warming to live alongside. I'm not sure that I can identify the point at which our love for each other, as partners, got rekindled.

Esther certainly had some very strong views about these issues and a big hand in this process.

For myself, I eventually found I couldn't resist falling right back in love with this woman who had stuck by her commitment to being Esther's parent with such resilience, humour and energy.

Nowadays we all live together in the same neighbourhood, in a house by the park and we mostly have a pretty good time, just making ourselves up as we go along. It is not always that peaceful at our house, but frankly it never was with two bossy, determined, Jewish women living together, and now that Esther is getting bigger we seem to have three bossy, determined Jewish woman living together …

We have a new Labour government in Britain these days, but they have not yet chosen to repeal clause 28, despite our very best efforts to persuade them to do so. Indeed, the British home secretary, Jack Straw, recently described children like our beautiful, gutsy daughter Esther as the 'Trophy' children of gay and lesbian couples who want it both ways. Well, that's not quite how we see it and I suppose we ought to continue to campaign against this law. The problem is that I'm not at all sure that I want to fight against this idea of 'pretended' families any longer. All in all, we've done a pretty good job of 'pretending' to be a family so far.

Perhaps we should campaign to keep clause 28, but turn the wording back to front. In this way, the British government and it's agencies would be prevented, by law, from promoting any definitions of what constitutes a 'real' family.

Then we could all be left to live our lives as best we could, just making ourselves up as we go along.

# 9

# Cummer Waltzing

## Being mothers together in adventurous and unconventional ways

by

Manja Visschedijk

*Just prior to the keynote session on alternative families taking place, Manja Visschedijk, spoke briefly about the beautiful quilt that was adorning the stage. Here is a copy of what she said.*

*Goeiemorgen allemaal, mijn naam is Manja Visschedijk en Ik wou graag deze bedoerde kleedt voorstellen. Ik heb het zelf gemaakd en het gaat over mijn familie.*

Good Morning everyone, I couldn't resist taking the rare opportunity of using my first language, Dutch! One of the things I have loved most about this conference has been hearing other languages spoken.

I acknowledge being on Kaurna land and that it is a privilege to be here.

I would like to take a few minutes to introduce you to my quilt. A few weeks ago I received the conference program and was hugely excited to read about this keynote celebrating alternative families. One of the things I did with that excitement was to email David Denborough about my quilt and to ask if it would be okay to bring it along. I was a bit worried about intruding and taking up space that belonged to this morning's speakers, but they have graciously included me and I thank them for that!

This is a story quilt and its name is 'Cummer Waltzing'. I made it for the grandchildren of our family – even though they haven't been born yet, and even if they aren't born from our own children. In the sewing of this quilt for our grandchildren I have experienced myself as 'legitimately familied' again, something I had been in danger of losing touch with as a result of some troubled times over the past few years.

So, the name of this quilt is Cummer Waltzing. I came across the word 'Cummer' about twenty years ago in the Oxford English Dictionary. It is an Old English word derived from two French words, 'Com' and 'Mere', meaning 'Co-mother'. I have taken it up to mean 'Being Mothers Together' and you can see that there are three circles in this central piece of the quilt which represent the three primary mothers of our family – Annie, Tikka and myself.

The word 'Waltzing' I took from an Australian song called 'Waltzing Matilda' which represents to me a spirit of adventure and rebellion against established and dominating ways.

So, Cummer Waltzing means Being Mothers Together in Adventurous and Unconventional Ways.

You will see if you look closely, the names of all the other people – and the furry friends – who have sustained and supported us over the years. It also has a date on it 1980-2000, to mark the twenty years since Annie and I first met and began to plot and dream our family into being.

The other two central pieces are for our children, Morgen, who is seventeen years of age and Gipsy, who is thirteen.

The remaining six pieces are called Amarant, Migration, Avalon, Change, Hope and Joy.

I made this quilt for our grandchildren because I want them to know some of the stories that make us a family. I imagine them climbing under this quilt at bedtime and asking for a story from one of these pieces.

*And when they do that I will tell them stories about love and how deeply and truly it flows between us, no matter whether we are connected through our hearts and by love, or our bodies and by blood.*

*I will them about how their grandmothers met and came to love one another.*

*I will tell them about their donors and how we came to meet them.*

*I will tell them about boy children and girl children and the politics of that.*

*I will tell them stories about loyalty and commitment and never giving up on our family.*

*I will tell them stories about Yowrie and Wallaga Lake and Gulaga mountain who sheltered and protected us.*

*I will tell them stories about picnics and parties and celebrations.*

*I will tell them stories about migration and how I learned from my own parents that it's possible to sail into uncharted waters and make a new and a good life there.*

*I will tell them stories about following your dreams and watching them blossom and grow. I will tell them about rainbow peoples and the spirits of change and hope and joy.*

*And I will tell them about a sister and a brother and how they give shape to each other and bring meaning and purpose and an immeasurable richness into the lives of all who know them.*

*I will tell them stories about coming here today and speaking about us to you.*

*I will tell them stories about how sometimes our family nearly became invisible, even to ourselves, and the magics that made us be seen again.*

*Like this magic of speaking and sharing and listening and honouring. This magic of making meaning in the spaces between us.*

*I invite you all to come and look at this quilt later and touch it and enjoy it and talk to each other about it – and feel free to speak to me about it too if you want to.*

# PART TWO

# *Talking about heterosexual dominance and homophobia*

This section provides a broader framework for considering some of the issues relevant to lesbian, gay and bisexual people within the therapy world.

# 10

# Heterosexual dominance in the world of therapy?

by

Daphne Hewson

## Bipolar labels

It is estimated that about 1 in 10 of us is homosexual. Presumably this means that 1 in 10 identify with the label of homosexual in terms of a bipolar split on sexuality. Another way of thinking about sexual orientation is in terms of a continuum. For example, Adrienne Rich (1980) suggests that we can describe a range of woman-identified experience (forms of intimacy and support between women) with only one end of the continuum representing a fully woman-centered identification in terms of both intimacy and sexuality. Many of those other 9 in 10 women are likely to identify themselves somewhere towards the fully woman-centered position, even if they do not choose sexual relationships with women.

This is an important concept, because it invites us to escape from the dominant bipolar notions of homosexual-heterosexual, and from the focus on the 'sexual' at the expense of 'intimacy'; it also allows an opening for sexual and intimacy preferences to be recognised as a choice, rather than the prescription of 'compulsory heterosexuality' (Rich 1980) which dominates in our society.

The problem with the concept, however, is that it tends to confound emotional and sexual forms of intimacy by placing them side-by-side on the same continuum. When discussing this confounding, my colleague, Corinne Roberts, suggested that it might be more helpful to conceptualise two continua, one based on emotional intimacy and another based on sexual interests and behaviours. Each continuum could range from a preference which is exclusively for one's own gender (homo), through various degrees of interest in both genders, to an exclusive preference for the other gender (hetero). Thus, the privilege and oppression of women who identify closely with the woman end of both continua (homo-intimacy and homo-sexuality) would not be attributed to women who identify somewhere towards 'homo-intimacy' but somewhere towards 'hetero-sexuality' in their sexual interests and practices.

Who would identify as totally 'hetero' on both continua? My guess is that few women would do so, because women have developed the opportunity to experience valued intimacy with other women in their family and friendship networks. Many have also had pleasurable experiences of touch and physical affection with other women. Men have not been so privileged. The dominant discourse on masculinity (which is heterosexual and homophobic-based), the limited opportunities for men to learn to value intimacy with other men, the common cultural taboo on touch between men (except for firm handshakes), and the cultural training for men to turn to women for their intimacy needs, all invite many men to identify closely with the 'hetero' end of both dimensions.

The purpose of this preamble is to suggest that it is possible to position oneself outside of the dominant assumption that there is one distinct group (heterosexuals) and another distinct group (homosexuals), and that it is, therefore, not necessary to identify on the 'them' or 'us' side of a gaping chasm. Although most of the paper addresses the impact of one's position on the homo/hetero sexuality continuum, it seems useful to start by posing questions concerning both continua:

- *Where would you presently place yourself on the homo/hetero intimacy continuum and on the homo/hetero sexuality (interest and practice) continuum?*
- *What experiences and training have contributed to these self-perceptions and practices?*
- *Do you experience any dysfunctions between your self-perceptions on the two continua? If so, how do these affect your life?*

**Acknowledging difference**

Despite the advantages of conceptualising a sexuality continuum, rather than bipolar labels, I recognise that it can sometimes be very helpful to highlight group distinctions. In fact, to minimise the differences in experience between publicly-identified heterosexuals and homosexuals can be a form of oppression.

For example, my friend, Jim, decided that he was sick of being 'in the closet' and that, despite the risks to his career as a school teacher, he would disclose to his colleagues. He disclosed during a meeting when they were all present. After an initial period of confusion, during which various people spoke about barely-related incidents, Jim repeated his disclosure and asked for comments. One of the women responded that she didn't see what the fuss was about. She said that she didn't see why homosexuals wanted to tell people about it. She thought the heterosexual custom of not commenting on one's sexual preferences was less intrusive and avoided discomfort for everyone. She added that she didn't judge people on their sexuality and that she didn't think anyone else did, so it didn't matter. Another woman responded 'So, would it be okay by you if the Principal thought that you were lesbian?' Suddenly sexuality mattered.

**Absence of attention**

The above example is a good illustration of the point that Kathleen Stacey (1993) makes when she quotes Card's (1992) comment that *Ignorance is not, strictly speaking, absence of knowledge: it is absence of attention* (p.45). The woman who thought that she believed that sexuality didn't matter was not ignorant of the oppression of homosexuals in our society, she simply hadn't previously been invited to pay attention to it. As soon as her attention was directed to the possible ramifications if she was disclosed as lesbian, her previously unrecognised knowledge was fully, and painfully, available to her. If she had chosen to attend to this opening further then more knowledge would have been quickly acquired.

Another example of absence of attention is a friend's recent experience when she was discussing the issue of touch with her male supervisor. She told him that a woman client had attempted to give her a hug at the end of a session in which they were working on the legacies of childhood sexual abuse. She had pulled back from the hug and was worried that the client might perceive this as rejection. The supervisor thought that she was creating, an unnecessary problem. He saw no reason why a female counsellor could not allow a hug from a female client after a successful session. She asked what he would have done. He replied that, as a man, he never touched young women clients. But he thought it was different for her.

The supervisor's response contains three examples of inattention to sexuality issues. Firstly, he seems to share with Queen Victoria a blindness to the possibility that women can be sexual with each other. Touch between women, even if they both identify as heterosexual, has the potential to be experienced as sexual and, thus, to be abusive in a therapeutic relationship.

Secondly, the supervisor seems to have assumed that the counsellor is heterosexual. Although she had not explicitly drawn his attention to her lesbian identity, the counsellor usually discusses it comfortably if given an opening. One's sexual identity is not a neutral factor in working with women, men, or families, and so it deserves attention in supervisory relationships. The absence of attention to her lesbian identity robbed this counsellor of the opportunity to develop her understanding of how it impacts on her work and how to address it in interactions with her clients.

Thirdly, women who are working on the legacies of sexual abuse are vulnerable to questioning their sexuality. Many heterosexually identified women tend to question their sexuality with men, and many lesbians tend to question whether the abuse 'caused' their homosexuality as a reaction against men. In the context of this questioning, intimacy and touch with a woman counsellor can have a significant meaning, especially when safety and trust legacies are being addressed in therapy. The absence of attention to the meaning that the hug had for the woman client robs her of the opportunity to explore this process in her healing. If the client has guessed that her counsellor is lesbian and/or is experiencing some attraction (transference?) towards her, then it seems particularly important to address the meaning of the hug, and the counsellor's withdrawal from it, in the context of the client's preferred narrative.

- *What might have been different if the supervisor had attended to the possibility of sexuality between women, or had recognised the counsellor's lesbian identity, or had asked some questions about the counsellor's thoughts about the meaning of the hug for her and for her client?*

**Some personal examples**

In my first ten years of work as a therapist I knowingly worked with only one homosexual client. The referring person told me that the client was lesbian and that she insisted that this be acknowledged. Thinking of myself as 'open-minded' (despite the fact that a shock treatment programme for homosexuals was operating just down the hall!), I tried to show acceptance of her sexuality by commenting in the first session, 'And I believe that you are homosexual?' It didn't come off with the flair I intended. My voice dropped and I stammered! She grinned mischievously and responded, 'What was that?' So I had to repeat my 'casual' question, much to my embarrassment.

I attempted to 'normalise' and 'accept' my client's sexuality by ignoring it and not asking questions about how it impacted on her life. Fortunately, she refused to accept this oppression. Over time, she desensitised me to some aspects of lesbian experience and educated me in ways to validate it in the therapy room. As I write that, I realise how it was another form of oppression. A client should not have to 'treat' her therapist's ignorance and homophobia.

And the learning did not generalise. I continued to be inattentive to sexuality with other clients, assuming (without realising that I was doing so) that every client I met was heterosexual.

The journey to my own lesbian identity was similarly hampered by absence of attention. I had a close woman friend whom I loved to be with. I thought of her often, dreamt about her, felt bereft if I didn't see her, and experienced greater intimacy with her than with anyone else in my life. But we were both heterosexual women and the possibility of lesbianism didn't enter my consciousness. If it had been suggested to me, I suspect I would have said that I couldn't be lesbian because I liked sex with men and had a reasonable marriage and two young children. My internalised model of a lesbian was someone who hated men, acted butch, and did not (could not?) mother children. I didn't know that I knew closet lesbians (even role models in the world of therapy) who were very different from that.

An unexpected event focussed my attention on sexuality. I rapidly moved from identifying as 'het' to identifying as lesbian, and started to allow myself to enjoy my lesbian self (this is probably not the place to share all the delightful details). Then I started to notice my homophobia. For example, I had previously been completely comfortable walking down the street arm-in-arm with women friends. Now I wondered if people were thinking that I was lesbian. I also had difficulty embracing the name 'dyke' which many lesbians have reclaimed for themselves (now I love the word).

A different form of inattention influenced my next stage. Since I had two preschool children and a conservative Christian family of origin, I assumed that it was easiest to keep my sexuality a secret. The stress of leaving the marriage, setting up shared parenting with the children's father across our two households, and dealing with family stress reactions, seemed like enough to handle. It took several years to realise that the option of invisibility is a dangerous onc. I couldn't have open relationships with women, so fear, secrecy and shame contributed to destroying my lover relationship with my friend. I couldn't talk freely about my sexuality with anyone but my lesbian friends, so my other friendships and family contacts became increasingly superficial. As the children grew older, I started to feel guilty that I was living a lie to them and wondered what would happen if they discovered my secret before I told them.

I wish Jo-Ann Kresten's (1988) article had been written by then. It would have allowed me to attend to the corner I was inadvertently painting myself into, and to come out much earlier than I did. She argues that:

> *... disclosure is important to the lesbian in order for her to counteract her tendency to internalize the homophobic message of society, in order for*

> *her to build authentic personal relationships with family members, and in order to avoid the pressure to form an increasingly closed system with her lover and other gay friends that is intensified by secrecy.* (p.119)

My memories of that time resonate with Jo-Ann Kresten's quote from Clark (1977) who says that:

> *Each time you pretend to be non-Gay when you are Gay, you give yourself a silent irrational message that it is wrong and bad to be the person you are.* (p.62)

The reasoning seems to be 'I want them to like and respect me, so I'll pretend to be the person they want me to be and then they'll like and respect the me I'm pretending to be'. This is a self-imposed punishment for being unacceptable within the dominant discourse, and only serves to strengthen the prescription that there is something bad or wrong with being who one is. If therapists intentionally or inadvertently collude with this self-imposed punishment, then does the punishment become therapist-imposed too?

Coming-out issues operate for all members of a homosexual's family. For example, when my 11 year old daughter was nine, she decided to tell some of her school friends that I am lesbian. They are all very interested in seeing me and my partner and asking questions about us. But they have chosen not to tell their parents. So she has a secret with them. My 14 year old son is out about me only to close family friends. He has decided not to 'subject himself to the problems he thinks he would experience if he told his school mates'. What influence are these secrets having on my children's internalisation of acceptable sexuality, or of their perceptions of the 'acceptability' of me and my partner? (And what do you call your lesbian mother's partner – your stepmother?)

Given the common assumption that we are all heterosexual until proven otherwise, a homosexual-identified person who wants to be out has to make constant decisions about how to do this. When you meet someone do you say, 'Hi, I'm Daf, and I'm lesbian'? Do you put it on the agenda for announcement at a staff meeting? Do you wear lavender clothes and lesbian earrings and hope that others know the code? Do you talk about 'my partner' and 'they' and hope that others notice these clues? Do you wait until someone asks about your husband or boyfriend and then create embarrassment for them by saying that 'he' is a 'she'? And how should clients inform their therapist? I think many try to do it by clues. But what are they supposed to do if their therapist misses the clues?

In my work as a therapist, I no longer have the problem of being 'a' heterosexual who does not notice homosexuality. Now I'm 'a' homosexual who has to decide whether or not to come out to my heterosexual clients. I always come out to therapists I am supervising, but I've taken the 'need to know' line with clients and disclosed only when sexuality has been a subject of therapy. I often wonder if this is another form of oppression, either for me (pretending to be who they think I am) or for them (being denied information which they might consider important in our work together). I'm interested in others' perspectives on this dilemma.

**A heterosexual questionnaire**

If you let someone know that you are gay or lesbian, then you are likely to be asked a number of 'well-meaning' questions about it. I started putting together a list of typical questions. Some of them were told to me by clients as ones they were asked by other therapists (leading them to find a lesbian therapist). I was intending to provide the list with a commentary on the underlying assumptions and point out how oppressive they are for gays and lesbians. But the commentary started to sound like a soap-box lecture, so I've switched the questions around. If you imagine a heterosexually-identified person being asked the questions, in therapy or by their family and friends, you'll be able to provide your own commentary.

1. *When did you first start to realise that you were heterosexual?*
2. *How did you know?*
3. *Are you sure ? Perhaps it's just a phase?*
4. *Did you fight the urge?*
5. *Have you sought help for it (I hear they can fix it with shock therapy if you're really motivated to get better)?*
6. *Were you sexually abused as a child?*

7. *Do you think it's because you went to a co-ed school?*
8. *Do you think it's because you had an unhappy homosexual relationship?*
9. *Is anyone else in your family heterosexual?*
10. *Are you providing your children with some good role models of homosexual families ?*
11. *What do you actually do in bed?*
12. *Even if you are 'that way', wouldn't it be fairer to your family to live a normal life as a homosexual?*
13. *Do you know that I still love you and think of you as normal?*
14. *I can accept that you are heterosexual, but don't you think it would be better not to tell your mother?*
15. *You and the children are welcome to come home for Christmas, but would you mind not bringing your partner?*
16. *We're happy to have you stay with us, but you do understand that we couldn't put you in the same* room?[1]
17. *Why do you have to flaunt it by touching each other in public?*
18. *For men: Are you a man-hater?* For women: *Are you misogynist?*
19. *Did your mother* (for women: *father) neglect you so that you need a woman (man) to mother (father) you as an adult?*
20. *All you need is a good '....' (with a person of your own gender). Why don't you try it?*

The purpose of this questionnaire is not to discourage therapists from asking clients anything about their homosexual identity or experience. On the contrary, these are important issues to be addressed. It is a myth that homosexual-identified persons are free of homophobia. When homophobia is an inevitable consequence of the dominant discourse, everyone is vulnerable to internalising it, especially those who have to live the day-by-day repercussions of being a member of the 'deviant' group.

Questions about how homosexuality influences a person's life and relationships, and their view of themselves, are likely to create openings for deconstructing heterosexual dominance in their lives and freeing them of vulnerability to homophobia and its associated shame. Not to ask such questions is to inadvertently exclude experiences which are fundamental to a person's identity and self-narrative.

**A Wish List – What would be different**

* *If all therapists advertised themselves as 'couple' therapists, rather than 'marital' therapists and there were 'Couple Centres' rather than 'Marriage Guidance' centres?*
* *If one of our international journals was called the Journal of Couple & Family Therapy?*
* *If no therapists made assumptions about a person's sexuality or the gender of their partner or the sexuality of the parents of their child clients?*
* *If all therapists recognised that, no matter whether clients label themselves as homosexual or heterosexual, they are each likely to vary in their position on both the homo/hetero intimacy continuum and the homo/hetero sexuality continuum, and that these positions influence their lived experience?*
* *If gays and lesbians didn't have to cover up social embarrassment when their therapist realises they had made an unjustified assumption about sexuality?*
* *If gay and lesbian clients never had to desensitise or educate their therapists about their lives?*
* *If no therapists ever tried to 'normalise' gay or lesbian clients by avoiding discussions of the impact of their sexuality on their lived experience?*
* *If gay and lesbian clients felt free to explore their internalised homophobia with their therapists without fearing that their sexual orientation would be questioned?*
* *If no therapists assumed sameness in the sexual behaviours and patterns of gay, lesbian, and heterosexual clients (for example, not using penis-based criteria for considering lesbian sexuality) ?*

* *If it was legally, occupationally and personally safe for all gay and lesbian therapists to come out to their colleagues? (and to their clients?)*
* *If therapists presenting at conferences or workshops sometimes discussed their work with homosexual couples and had a consistent pattern of labelling the sexuality of all couples, not just 'homosexual couples'?*
* *If all therapists who have not identified about 1 in 10 of their adult clients as homosexual, asked themselves 'Why'?*
* *If all therapists recognised that the ending of a gay or lesbian relationship has the same potential importance to each partner and to their children as the ending of a heterosexual marriage?*
* *If all therapists acknowledged to children and adolescents who have gay or lesbian parents that this influences their lives, rather than having it 'normalised'?*
* *If the role of the non-biological parent in gay and lesbian couples was fully acknowledged and appreciated by all therapists (and by the law)?*
* *If no therapists were affected by the dominant discourse that gay men are in some way responsible for AIDS?*
* *If all therapists asked gay clients about the impact on their life and their relationships of their losses of friends and lovers in the AIDS epidemic?*

**Acknowledgement**

Many thanks to Mary Dawson for her support and helpful comments during the preparation of this paper.

# 11

# The power of language

by

Suzy Stiles

*Homophobia, heterosexism* and *heterosexual dominance* – what's the difference? Does it matter anyway? Navigating the sometimes stormy and always changing sea of language is not easy. But for those of us who are impatient for change, the journey can be both a creative and a necessary adventure.

Over the last 20 years, feminists, anti-racists and others have restated an old truth – language is power. The terminology of the powerful routinely demeans the powerless (women are 'girls', men of colour are 'boys'). Women, people of colour and others accustomed to the sharp end of belittling or abusive language have therefore argued for words which reflect the choice of people to describe themselves.

These new ways of thinking about language have of course been pilloried by those who love to condemn what they call 'political correctness'. It provides endless creative fun for the ostrich defenders of the status quo, who miss the point with their 'politically correct' parodies ('Snow Unpigmented and the Seven Differently Sized Male Persons' is the most recent jibe I've seen).

Less fun for writers and editors in the media circus is the concept of 'political awareness', a life-affirming faculty which employs heart and mind and spirit. It is this, not political correctness, which can understand and discriminate between offensive, appropriate, respectful and silly language.

**All the world's queer ...**

The debates around language are alive and well in queer politics, as elsewhere. In 1990s North America, the word *queer* has been reclaimed and is the new *bon mot* for the urban, young, activist and academic.

This practice of reclamation is not new. When I was younger it felt daring and politically fashionable to call ourselves *dykes. Faggot,* a term of abuse originating when gay men were used like faggots to fuel the flames which burnt witches in medieval Europe, is now claimed with pride by gay men. We can also deduce from the definitions of 'witchlike' behaviour which were used at the time that the 'witches' themselves were probably often lesbians.

*Queer* as a term has the advantage of being inclusive of all non-dominant sexualities, and avoids the cumbersomeness of having to repeatedly list lesbians, gay men, bisexuals and transsexuals.

It avoids the fraught term 'gay', which some would argue has reached its use-by date. (Does *gay* include women? A murky question which has seen many groups over the last five to ten years change their names to include the words *Lesbian and Gay).* It also avoids problematic categorisation, and is therefore preferred by those who argue that sexuality should be understood as a spectrum, not a finite category.

However, in Australia *queer* is not widely recognised beyond inner city politics and the world of urban chic and many people in the lesbian and gay communities would not identify as queer.

**The love that dares to speak its name**

The importance of creating a language that describes our diverse non-heterosexual identities should not be underestimated. The oppression of gay men and lesbians in the West has been unique in the level of silence that surrounded us. It's not just that the words were not of our own choosing – they hardly existed, and certainly weren't allowed to be spoken. For lesbians in particular, this linguistic absence encouraged those who, like Queen Victoria, denied our very existence.

This is why visibility is so crucial an act for lesbians and gay men – and why we have to 'go on about it'. To adapt an old feminist adage: *The power of heterosexual dominance is the silence of the queer.*

Finding the language to describe oppression is an act of power as important as finding words to describe our own sense of self. The use of the term patriarchy, for example, shifted the whole territory on which 'the Women's Question' was debated.

**Homophobia**

The term *homophobia* has been used for the last 30 years to cover all manner of hatred, discrimination and bigotry towards gay men and lesbians. It has been a useful tool in the attempts of lesbian and gay activists to move the locus of evil from the object of hatred to the perpetrator of hate. The term articulates the belief that prejudice, not homosexuality, is the problem.

However, like the word *homosexual,* it is arguably problematic. For most people the image conjured up by both words is that of gay men.

In fact, the root of both is *homos,* Greek for equal or same, not *homo,* Latin for man – but this unfortunately doesn't change popular perception, and the inherent exclusion of lesbians.

For others, *phobia* seems inappropriate, more reminiscent of the fear of spiders than of the hatred and contempt that causes virulent verbal attacks or gay bashing.

Another difficulty is that *homophobia* sounds like *homosexuality.* It therefore doesn't do much to point the finger towards dominant heterosexuality as the source of the problem, or towards those who benefit from and have the upper hand in perpetuating heterosexuality as naturally superior.

In addition, *homophobia* is often used in a context which suggests that the problem belongs to a particular, especially bigoted individuals or groups. Unlike the concept of *heterosexual dominance,* it does not encourage a vision of the whole system which perpetuates heterosexuality as the naturally 'right' and desirable mode.

**Heterosexism or heterosexual dominance?**

The concept of heterosexism has its roots in feminist thought, and in particular we owe much to that powerful poet and radical thinker, Audre Lorde. In *Sister Outsider* she articulates the problem as *a belief in the inherent superiority of one pattern of loving over all others, and thereby its right to dominance.*

More recently, Joseph Neilsen (1990) provided the following useful analysis:

> *Heterosexism is the continual promotion by major social institutions of heterosexuality and the simultaneous subordination of all other lifestyles (that is, gay, lesbian and bisexual). It is based on unfounded prejudice, just as racism and sexism are. When our institutions knowingly or unknowingly perpetuate these prejudices and intentionally or unintentionally act on them, heterosexism is at work.*
>
> *Heterosexism is not limited to institutional oppression. Individual acts of heterosexism occur when individuals discriminate and institutions passively allow or foster the continuation of such discrimination. Heterosexism manifests itself in blatant discrimination against gays and lesbians, as well as in more subtle forms of exclusion or lack of recognition.*
>
> *Heterosexism is alive when individuals refuse to rent to gays or lesbians, when the military discharges someone for homosexual behaviour or the mere suspicion of being homosexual, and when governments prohibit gays and lesbians from marrying legally.*
>
> *Heterosexism also works in more subtle ways, as when television programs and advertisements show only heterosexual couples, when mainstream media under report gay and lesbian events ... and when obituaries fail to acknowledge the life partners of gay men and lesbians.*

We may see ourselves as tolerant, kind and opposed to all forms of discrimination, and still find ourselves being subtly or perhaps even blatantly heterosexist. Lesbians and gay men aren't magically exempt either, although it's harder for us not to notice when we're the ones being excluded.

If you sit and think for a bit, it won't be hard to remember a time when you've done a bit of inadvertent exclusion or made an assumption. Have you ever assumed a colleague's partner is the opposite sex? Asked whether your friend's daughter has a boyfriend yet? The list goes on and on.

Finally we come to *heterosexual dominance.* Many prefer this term to *heterosexism,* which is actually a misnomer for something that would more accurately be called *sexual orientationism,* that is, assigning a superior value to a single sexual orientation (wait til the PC bashers get a hold of that one!).

*Heterosexual dominance,* although an unwieldy mouthful unlikely to catch on in the school playground, has the advantage of pinpointing the process whereby heterosexuality is not only assigned superior value, but dominates and is actively asserted over all others. It refers to a system in which inequities of power are produced and maintained, and helps create an understanding that it is this systematised inequity that has to be challenged if we are to create any real change. It's not just about being nice to gay men and lesbians, though the rhetoric of this, the International Year for Tolerance, might lead you to think so.

If you're left wondering which terms to use, I'd suggest all three. I do. Yes, *homophobia* has a shelf life, but it's a term that's much more readily understood than *heterosexism* or *heterosexual dominance* (which has been confused with the top position in heterosexual SM sex!).

*Homophobia* also for me comes closer to expressing the virulent contempt, violence, or personal attacks I have experienced in my life. *Heterosexual dominance* is somehow too conceptual a term to catch the essence of being spat at in the face, or having fires lit on your doorstep, or reading graffiti down your street that says 'Get out you AIDS fuckers – gay men and lesbians are killing our kids!'

Having said that, the terms *heterosexism* and *heterosexual dominance* will be crucial in attacking the power systems which fuel this sort of homophobia. Without implicating all the structures of heterosexuality we cannot creat[illegible]sting political and social change. So until someone comes up with something catchier than *heterosexual dominance,* I'm practising getting my tongue round it!

# 12

# Speaking out from the dominant position

by

Chris McLean

Until quite recently, I have always thought of myself as heterosexual, without questioning what that really meant. I acknowledged that I belonged 'to a dominant and oppressive masculine culture, and spent time thinking about issues of gender and race. I recognised that my position of privilege brought with it ethical dilemmas. How could I work to dismantle an unjust system from which I simultaneously benefited? How could I know whether my efforts to produce change were not simply reproducing dominant culture in ways that were invisible to me? However, I had certainly never thought of myself as heterosexually dominant!

In grappling with this question I have been lucky enough to be included in invitations from some lesbian women and gay men to look at my participation in the dominant culture of heterosexism. I have found it relatively easy to see heterosexual dominance at work in the society at large, and to see it in the actions and attitudes of people around me. I have, however, found it quite difficult to see in myself.

I know that I am not alone in this. For some reason, many people from the dominant culture who are genuinely engaged in challenging injustice in many areas of life are strangely ignorant of, and silent about, the oppression experienced by their gay and lesbian brothers and sisters.

This article is intended to explore why this is so, and to ask what responsibilities members of the dominant heterosexual culture have to challenge this situation. In order to be able to write it, I have talked with and interviewed a number of straight men and women working in a variety of ways within the 'helping professions'. They have all been engaged for some time in exploring issues of heterosexual dominance with gay and lesbian colleagues.

The first thing to be clear about is that there is a problem! Lesbians and gay men are telling us this very clearly, but most straight people simply don't want to know about it. The 'problem' ranges from the obvious example of homophobic violence, to the more insidious expressions such as the total absence of positive gay and lesbian images in our mainstream public media. This is not the place to go into any detail of what gay men and lesbians experience on a daily basis. It is enough to say that this injustice exists, it is not minor, and that if we have an ethical commitment to social change, we cannot go on ignoring it. Ignorance is not an excuse, it is part of the problem!

The very invisibility of the issue needs careful examination. Gay and lesbian colleagues, friends and acquaintances who feel safe enough to relate their pain to us or challenge us will probably be from the same class and racial background, and often of the same gender. They may have professional qualifications, good incomes and seem 'just like us'. How can they regard themselves as oppressed? How can they justify time being spent on their concerns when we are already working so hard with people who are obviously in crisis?

We need to remember that the invisibility of oppression does not mean that it does not exist. Gay men and lesbians have put enormous amounts of effort into remaining invisible as a matter of survival. To use this invisibility to justify non-action is cruelly unjust. Gays and lesbians also take on an almost overwhelming responsibility for anticipating possible outcomes of any interaction with straight people, dealing with their responses, both good and bad, and following through the ongoing consequences of these interactions.

In any situation where a dominant and a marginalised culture meet, it is useful to remind ourselves that the best judges of whether an injustice has occurred are people in a marginalised position. Our very membership of the dominant group means that we will be unable to see many of the injustices which are so glaringly obvious to those who are affected by them every day of their lives.

It seems to me that the first responsibility we have is to educate ourselves about the realities of the world we live in. There is a vibrant gay and lesbian literature of which most straight people (including me) know little. In my own academic area of gender and history, many of the major works are written by gay and lesbian scholars. They are also developing many of the most exciting new theoretical understandings of sexuality, ethics, and popular culture. However, I must admit that my knowledge of these writings barely scratches the surface. This can only have come from some sense that the 'gay experience' is 'other'[1] and marginal to the 'real business' of academic understanding.

Similarly, we need to be wary of simplistic generalisations. In a society which prioritises male experience, talking about 'gay issues' tends to hide the fact that lesbian experience is different from that of gay men. Even talking about 'gay and lesbian issues' without acknowledging those differences can reinforce the invisibility so often experienced by lesbians. Heterosexual people should not assume that if they deal with gay men's issues they will automatically understand lesbian issues as well.

There is a whole world 'out there' in which gay men and lesbians are grappling with the suffering and injustices of HIV/AIDS, with no recognition from dominant culture. Three times as many men have died from AIDS as died in the Vietnam War - but where are the mass movements, marches and demands for action that emerged from the whole community in response to that situation? It has been said that a form of genocide is taking place in our very midst, and we go on as if nothing were happening.

There is a great need for us all to recognise and celebrate the achievements of the gay and lesbian communities. For example, we need to publicly acknowledge their contribution to dealing with HIV/AIDS. The Australian government basks in the international recognition of its leading place in HIV/AIDS prevention policies, but fails to mention that without the concerted action of gays and lesbians these policies would never have been introduced.

Similarly, public events such as the Mardi Gras are important antidotes to the invisibility of gay and lesbian issues and lives. As the Mardi Gras becomes more and more popular and accepted we should not forget that it initially faced fierce police repression and overwhelming public hostility.

In contrast to the non-action and indifference of most straight people to issues of homophobia, many gay and lesbian social workers, teachers, therapists (etc, etc) are making major contributions to the lives of straight people, while having to hide the source of much of their energy and commitment.

As well as educating ourselves about what is happening 'out there', we need to look at ourselves and recognise how the invisibility of heterosexual dominance is maintained in our own lives. It came as quite a shock to me recently to realise that I had constructed a major work of exclusion within my own friendships. I pride myself on my close male friendships. I talk to my men friends about anything and everything - or so I thought. We talk about relationships and share hopes and excitements as well as griefs and fears. Yet never once had the question of same-sex attraction been raised.

When I finally mentioned this to a long-time friend, he told me that he has had as many relationships with men as with women. I thought I knew him well, yet I never knew about an important part of who he is. I am now faced with renegotiating the boundaries of unquestioned relationships. What is it OK to say? What is it OK to ask? How many of my taken-for-granted knowledges are based on ignorance and silence?

To me this is symbolic of our whole society. Injustice is maintained, not so much by evil exploiters, but by the mass of 'good' people who have the privilege of being able to close their eyes and ears to the injustices all around them, because these injustices do not impact directly on them. This silence is then perpetuated by a system that discourages anyone from raising these issues.

On the other hand, gays and lesbians are continuously hyper-aware of our responses to any mention of these issues. Something we say might, to us, be simply flippant, but to our gay and lesbian acquaintances or friends it is a sign of how much we can be trusted.

Once we start to become aware of this and make efforts to find out more, we are faced with another dilemma. How can we take responsibility for challenging heterosexual dominance when we encounter it in our workplaces, in our families, and amongst our friends and acquaintances? This can be a very difficult process, confronting us with a range of dilemmas.

There is often a concern that gays and lesbians may not want straight people to speak up on these issues, particularly if it seems that straight people are trying to speak on their behalf. I have sometimes worried that it might be seen as presumptuous to speak out at all, and somehow to be denying the capacity of people from the marginalised position to speak for themselves. However, in all the conversations I have had with lesbians and gay men who are interested in the possibility of partnership with heterosexuals, there has been a very clear message to us: Gay men and lesbians definitely want straight people to challenge the homophobia of straight culture - however, the question of motivation is very important. We need to be clear why we, as heterosexual people, are involving ourselves in this area. If we are doing so simply to help others, we are effectively distancing ourselves from the issue and reinforcing our dominant position.

We need to find ways of speaking that make it clear that we are also speaking for ourselves. For myself, I have increasingly realised how much my experience of my body, my sexuality and my friendships with men and women are limited by the prescriptions of heterosexual culture. I have a longing for a deeper sense of connection and community, as well as a greater sense of freedom in my experience of myself. I am increasingly convinced that this is impossible without challenging the dominant culture of heterosexuality.

A number of people I spoke to talked about their desire to raise issues of heterosexual dominance in a tactful way. They did not want to look as if they were claiming the moral high ground and preaching to people they considered ignorant or misguided. There was a recognition of how important it is to find ways of speaking personally about issues, so that the speaker is not polarising a situation into 'goodies' and 'baddies', but acknowledging their own place within dominant culture. We need to find ways of accepting responsibility without being paralysed by a sense of blame. There are often very few opportunities for people to learn about these issues; and if we have had such opportunities, that is itself a privilege, and does not place us outside of our own culture.

Confronting people with their 'mistakes' in an aggressive way is extremely unlikely to be effective. I am talking here about action taken by members of the dominant culture - members of marginalised groups certainly have no responsibility for raising issues tactfully.

However, my experience, and that of the people I interviewed, has been that we have been treated with kindness and consideration by gay and lesbian colleagues when we have caused them pain through our own unconscious hetero-sexism. If we have been treated so thoughtfully ourselves, it would be profoundly dishonouring to treat others of our own group any differently. On a number of occasions it has been made quite clear to us that what gay men and lesbians really want is for us to 'hang in' with our straight colleagues, friends and acquaintances - not to write them off or give up on them because it seems too difficult to reach a shared understanding.

One woman I interviewed said how helpful she found it to *'carry community around in [her] head and heart'.* What she meant by this was that, if she tries to speak on issues of heterosexual dominance simply as an isolated individual, it often seems just too difficult. However, having made the effort to develop a network of like-minded people with whom she is exploring these issues, she can imagine them there with her when she needs to take action, and feels much more able to act.

In another interview, a woman spoke about her dilemmas of not knowing whether to speak up in public situations. She dealt with this by personally approaching lesbian women she knew afterwards and speaking of her dilemma. She has found this to be a powerful way of gaining a greater understanding of the issues, and a way of gaining greater confidence in her own judgement.

This speaks clearly of the need for straight people to develop links with gay men and lesbians. Without this it is impossible to know whether our well-intentioned efforts are simply reproducing dominant culture in ways that are invisible to us.

Similarly, a man spoke of confronting his fear of being labelled homosexual if he spoke out on these issues. He recognised that this was itself a product of his own homophobia. However, this is a very powerful part of dominant male culture, and it can be very difficult to deal with, particularly in isolation. This man has found that developing relationships with gay men and lesbians, as well as developing a community of straight people who regard these issues as important, is the only way of ensuring that he does not end up silenced or giving up.

As far as the workplace is concerned, this article is not intended to be a 'how-to' guide to practical measures one could take to make one's services appropriate to gay and lesbian clients; or how to create a safer and more inclusive environment for gay and lesbian co-workers.

There are, however, lots of practical things to be done. These include looking at the images which adorn our waiting room walls, and the magazines on the waiting room tables. How many images of gay men and lesbians do we see? How comfortable would gay men and lesbians feel in such an environment?

What about the wording of our forms and our interview questions? Do they assume heterosexual partners, for example? Do they speak of married and de facto relationships, or of partnerships and relationships? What about the conversations in the staff room at lunch time? Would gay or lesbian colleagues feel safe to talk about what they had done with their partners on the weekend? Would they feel safe to talk about a friend or partner dying of AIDS?

These are some of the questions we all need to be looking at. No article can answer them. The only answer is to find ways of entering into equitable partnerships with gay men and lesbians, to listen and then to take action. The opportunities are there if only we are willing to take them up.

# 13

# Who Cares?

## Institutional barriers to health care for lesbian, gay and bisexual persons

by

Michele J. Eliason[1]

a review by

David Denborough

Throughout the pages of this book, Michele Eliason, as a psychologist and a nurse, invites us as health professionals to consider the complicity of the health professions in the marginalisation of lesbian, gay and bisexual people, and to explore practical acts that will contribute to removing the institutional barriers that still exist. It is a thoughtful and moving book which begins with considerations of history.

## A consciousness of history

Eliason begins with an exposé of how the history of bisexual, lesbian, gay people's struggle is interwoven with that of the history of the health professions:

> *The word* homosexual *first appeared in the medical literature in 1869, and referred to a form of mental illness or deviant sexuality (an abnormal and excessive interest in people of the same sex). The term* heterosexual *appeared in the United States in a medical journal in 1892, and also originally referred to a mental illness – an abnormal and excessive interest in people of the other sex.* (Eliason 1996, p.18)

Although the terms *homosexual* and *heterosexual* may both have been terms of pathology for a short time, it was not long before this changed. Throughout the early years of sexology and psychology most research speculated on the origins of homosexuality, but rarely upon the origins of heterosexuality[2]. The idea was quickly advanced that *homosexuality needed explanation, but that heterosexuality did not; that heterosexuality was the norm and that homosexuality constituted the abnormal.* (Ibid)

The increased attention given to people with same-sex desires by the medical and health care professions led to enormous harm. Eliason describes how the health professions over the last two hundred years labelled homosexuality as a mental illness and then proceeded to develop and use a variety of treatments to 'cure' it. These had devastating effects:

> *Among the treatments are surgical measures: castration, hysterectomy, and vasectomy. In the 1800s, surgical removal of the ovaries and of the clitoris are discussed as a 'cure' for various forms of female 'erotomania', including, it seems, Lesbianism. Lobotomy was performed as late as 1951. A variety of drug therapies have been employed, including the administration of hormones, LSD, sexual stimulants, and sexual depressants. Hypnosis, used on Gay people in America as early as 1899, was still being used to treat such 'deviant behaviours' in 1967. Other documented 'cures' are shock therapy, both electrical and chemical; aversion therapy, employing nausea-inducing drugs, electric shock, and/or negative verbal suggestion; and a type of behaviour therapy called 'sensitization' intended to increase heterosexual arousal.*

*Often homosexuals have been the subject of Freudian psychoanalysis and other varieties of individual and group psychotherapy.* (Katz 1992 in Eliason 1996, pp.23-24)

Eliason also writes of the many gay, lesbian, and bisexual people who have been forcibly incarcerated in mental institutions and treated without their consent. Although experiences of forced treatment or incarceration occur less frequently to adults today, Eliason points out that young bisexual, lesbian and gay people are still vulnerable to being committed to institutions and/or treatments by their parents. The legacies of abusive histories live on:

*These negative experiences, coupled with the misuse of research to promote or perpetuate discrimination, led to a generalised distrust of medicine and health care institutions in general in many lesbian, gay, and bisexual people. The legacy left by early psychiatrists, and maintained by prejudiced health care providers today, constitutes a major barrier to quality health care in the 1990s.*[3] (Eliason 1996, p.24)

## Resistance

Ironically, the creation of the term *homosexual* by psychiatrists of the late nineteenth century also had positive effects, as Eliason (1996) describes: *The increased attention given to people with same-sex desires created a forum for them to learn about others with similar feeling, and allowed them to establish an identity based on that similarity* (p.23). This formation of a collective identity was the precursor to what became the gay liberation movement of the 1970s. The removal of homosexuality from the Diagnostic and Statistical Manual of Mental Disorders (DSM) in 1973 is among the many achievements of this movement.[4]

Communities of lesbian, gay and bisexual people have created their own understandings of their lives and their own cultures within which to live. They have also deconstructed the history and origins of thinking of the health professions which once placed them under observation. The gaze has been reversed![5] By tracing the history of the psychological and health professions, Eliason invites us as contemporary health professionals to acknowledge the legacies of our past and to ask more of ourselves in our current practice. What do these histories mean for us as health professionals? How do they speak to us differently depending upon whether we are gay, bisexual, lesbian, or straight? What actions can we take to remove the current institutional barriers to lesbian, gay and bisexual people accessing respectful health care?

## Invitations to action

Eliason goes on to focus on a number of areas in which health professionals can take action.

### *(i) Acknowledgment of gay, lesbian and bisexual families*

> *Health care providers have a responsibility to learn about lesbian and gay families, because they can have a major impact on these family units, depending on their attitudes.* (Ibid p.105)

Eliason goes on to explore the realities of gay, lesbian and bisexual families[6]. She describes in vivid terms the rights which these families are denied and the real implications of this. One man describes a situation in which their partner was unable to visit him in hospital in a time of a life-and-death crisis. A woman describes the effects of living with the knowledge that if her lesbian partner dies she is likely to lose custody of their child as she is not the child's biological mother.

Acknowledging the realities of alternative families brings a different focus to the work of health professionals. For a start it leads to alternative questions, processes and paperwork to those which assume heterosexuality. Eliason gives examples of alternative questions for workers to ask: *Instead of the usual marital status question, ask questions such as: With whom do you live? Who is important to you? Do you live with your sexual partner?* (p.185) She also provides examples of alternative intake forms which do not assume heterosexuality.

Acknowledging alternative families can also enable health professionals to be open to accessing support from those closest to their client, and asking different questions that are free from heterosexist assumptions, such as: *Will the client have a supportive partner, family of origin, family of creation, or community to foster recovery?* (p.104)

In situations where this support may not exist, Eliason writes of how health professionals need to know how to access (where possible) confidential counselling by gay / bisexual / lesbian affirmative professionals, support groups, organisations, as well as supportive physicians, lawyers and religious leaders.

Taking seriously the experiences of lesbian, gay and bisexual families also involves learning about ways of protecting these families from the homophobia and heterosexual dominance of the broader society:

> *To protect their relationships, lesbian, gay and bisexual families need several kinds of legal documents such as wills and power of attorney for finances and health care. Health care providers need to be skilled at ... advising couples on how to protect their relationships, particularly when one of the couple has a chronic illness, or when child custody is threatened.* (p.104)

In her writing, Eliason opens up the door to a whole territory of responsibilities for health professionals in relation to bisexual, gay and lesbian people.

***(ii) Disclosure of sexual identity to health care providers***

> *Next to disclosure of sexual identity to parents, disclosure to a health care provider can be one of the most stressful events in a lesbian, gay or bisexual person's life.* (p.91)

This startling quote introduces the reader to the complexities involved for lesbian, gay and bisexual people in thinking through whether they ought to speak of their sexual identity with health professionals. What would occur if all health professionals put in the same degree of thoughtfulness into how to make their workplace an equitable and respectful place for bisexual, lesbian and gay people? Reading of the ways in which gay, bisexual and lesbian people seek out supportive services, scan the setting for any signs of acceptance, and carefully note the response of health professionals if and when they do speak of their sexuality, is a powerful invitation to the reader to consider their own practices and workplace. Eliason makes it clear that we as health professionals have responsibilities not only to ensure that those who consult with us are in a position to speak of their sexuality, but also to consider our colleagues who may be gay, bisexual or lesbian.

***(iii) Violence and same-sex couples***

*Virtually all openly lesbian, gay or bisexual people have experienced some form of victimisation, such as verbal abuse, threats, being chased or followed, or being spat on. Gay-bashing is physical violence directed at a person solely on the basis of the individual's perceived sexual orientation, and affects about 20% of lesbian, gay and bisexual people in their lifetimes.* (p.93)

With violence and overt discrimination so common, Eliason writes of how health workers have a responsibility to be open to exploring the effects of this harassment in ways that avoid blaming the victim, that locate the violence in the broader context of homophobia to decrease self-blame, and that involve significant others into the healing process. She also writes of the importance of domestic violence workers to be aware of same-sex domestic violence and to develop respectful ways of responding to it.

***(iv) HIV/AIDS***

For heterosexual health professionals who have not been involved in responding to the HIV/AIDS crisis, the experience of AIDS on the gay, lesbian and bisexual world can be impossible to understand. And yet, according to Eliason, is it their responsibility to try:

*I learned I was HIV positive in 1987. I've probably been seropositive for longer than that. I've outlasted my lovers, my friends, some of my exes, my tricks, my relatives, even some of the queens I couldn't stand. I've outlasted our doctor. I've even outlasted the guilt of still being alive and healthy. It's funny. There is no satisfaction in that word: outlasted. There is no satisfaction in living longer than friends and loved ones. No catharsis crying at yet another memorial service. I don't go to them any more. The miracle of survival. Survival is a spot between the rock of guilt and the hard place of memory.* (Robert Vasquez-Pacheco in Eliason 1996, p.188)

Various quotes from people living with AIDS help to bring home to readers the realities of HIV/AIDS. Eliason also points out that addressing health professionals' AIDS-related stigma is a crucial concern: *AIDS is one of the few diseases whereby some health care providers assign blame, and distinguish among 'guilty' versus 'innocent' victims* (p.207). According to Eliason, not only must we as health professionals explore our fears and attitudes in relation to HIV/AIDS, but the AIDS epidemic also demands of us to revise our attitudes to speaking about sexual practices. She provides some practical suggestions so that questions about sexuality do not assume heterosexuality:

- *Regarding sexual activity, health care providers could ask:*
  *Do you practice safe sex with all your partners?*
  *What precautions do you use?*
- *Use specific terms like oral sex, vaginal sex, and anal sex instead of the vague 'sex' or 'intercourse'.* (p.185)

***(v) Challenging homophobia and heterosexual dominance***

> *Heterosexism is so deeply embedded in health care systems that it will require major efforts to ferret it out ... in hospital admission and health history forms, in the interview formats used by many health care providers that assume heterosexuality, in the educational pamphlets in clinics and waiting rooms, in the requirements for some procedures such as artificial insemination, in visiting hours policies, and in health care decision making and information sharing.* (p.214)

Homophobia and heterosexual dominance have enormous consequences on the lives of lesbian, gay and bisexual people who consult with us. An awareness of the effects and tactics of homophobia and heterosexual dominance allows us as health professionals to resist individualising and pathologising problems experienced by bisexual lesbian and gay people and to instead acknowledge their broader context.

Eliason describes how finding ways to free our workplaces from the effects of heterosexual dominance, and ways of changing worker attitudes are the responsibilities of all health professionals. Her examples of workplace situations make it clear that it is particularly up to heterosexual health workers to speak up on issues of heterosexism, as for them the risks of speaking up are far less.

Whether we work with children, adults, elderly persons, people with disabilities, mental health, in an institution or in private practice, these are issues relevant to us all. As Eliason describes, the chances are we all work and interact with bisexual, lesbian and gay people whether we know it or not.

## Asking questions of ourselves

Michele Eliason's book ends with the following quote from Audre Lorde, an African American lesbian poet and activist who died of breast cancer in 1992. Soon after her diagnosis and mastectomy in 1977, she wrote:

> *I have come to believe over and over again that what is most important to me must be spoken, made verbal and shared, even at the risk of having it bruised or misunderstood. That the speaking profits me, beyond any other effect ... In becoming forcibly and essentially aware of my mortality, and of what I wished and wanted for my life, however short it might be, priorities and omissions became strongly etched in a merciless light and what I most regretted were my silences. Of what had I ever been afraid? ... My silences had not protected me. Your silence will not protect you ... What are the words you do not yet have? What do you need to say? What are the tyrannies you swallow day by day and attempt to make your own, until you will sicken and die of them, still in silence. Perhaps for some of you here today, I am the face of one of your fears. Because I am woman, because I am black, because I am lesbian, because I am myself, a black woman warrior poet doing my work, come to ask you, are you doing yours?* (Audre Lorde in Eliason 1996, p.234)

Michele Eliason seems to be asking similar questions: Are we doing our work? Are we taking up our responsibilities as health professionals to redress the injustices of our professions' history? Are we taking the steps required to build health care practices and workplaces that are honouring of families, love and desire in whatever shape they evolve? Are we standing by as lesbian, gay and bisexual people's realities continue to go unspoken and unnoticed? Or are we taking action?

## Notes

1. *Who Cares? Institutional barriers to health care for lesbian, gay and bisexual persons*, by Michele J. Eliason, was published in 1996 by the National League of Nursing, New York, NY 10014.

2. Eliason points out that Freud's work was an exception to this exclusive focus on the origins of homosexuality. Although much psychoanalysis was negative about homosexuality, she writes 'this idea did not stem directly from Freud' (p.19). She goes to quote a letter which Freud wrote to a woman who was asking for help with her son, in which he writes: *Many highly respectable individuals of ancient and modern times have been homosexuals, several of the greatest men among them (Plato, Michelangelo, Leonardo da Vinci, etc). It is a great injustice to persecute homosexuality as a crime and a cruelty too ... By asking me if I can help, you mean, I suppose, if I can abolish homosexuality and make normal* (sic) *heterosexuality take its place. The answer is, in a general way, we cannot promise to achieve it.* (Freud [1935] in Katz 1983, p.506)

3. The legacy of these histories lives on in the many 'reparative' therapies to 'cure' homosexuality that are still on offer.

4. The DSM did retain a diagnosis referred to as 'Egodystonic Homosexuality,' which was used for the person who was unhappy with her/his sexual identity and wished to change. Eliason quotes MacDonald (1976) who noted that, before 1973, one was sick if she/he liked being homosexual, but after 1973, one was sick only if she/he did not like being homosexual! In 1986 this diagnosis was also removed from the DSM.

5. For a thorough and detailed critique of the role of psychology within the lesbian community see: *Changing Our Minds: Lesbian feminism and psychology,* by Celia Kitzinger & Rachel Perkins (1993), New York: New York University Press.

6. Eliason writes of the complexities of bisexual families: *If a bisexual person is in a relationship with a person of the other sex, that relationship appears to be heterosexual, carries all the privileges of heterosexuality, but renders the bisexuality of one or both of the partners invisible. When a bisexual person is in a -relationship with someone of the same sex, the relationship is treated as a gay or lesbian union, again erasing the bisexuality of one or both partners.* (p.82)

# PART THREE

# *Talking amongst ourselves*

Finding ways to talk with each other, to facilitate community conversations on the issues that can so easily divide, is one of the greatest challenges facing any marginalised community. Here, Paul Browde and Murray Nossel offer a most beautiful example of what it means to talk amongst ourselves.

# 14

# Friendship and community in the age of HIV

by

Paul Browde & Murray Nossel

*We are white South African men who live in New York City. We are gay. We are privileged to have the opportunity to tell our stories. We dedicate this talk to all people who are not free to tell their stories and to be heard.*

***Murray:*** There are magical places in the world. Places where you can feel yourself growing. Places where you know you are learning.

***Paul:*** We share a very special place in the world. It is called Ravina. Ravina is 30 acres of land on a mountain in the woods, overlooking the Delaware River, two and a half hours north of New York City. On the land there is a large house, a cottage and a bungalow. The three houses were built in the early part of the 20th century. The property is surrounded by a sixty year old, 700 foot hand-built stone wall. A stream runs down from the mountain, over the land and into the river. On weekends, and whenever else it's possible, our New York City community moves up to Ravina. Our community consists of Murray and his partner David, my partner Simon and me, our friend Natalie, and our friend Craig.

In summer at Ravina, we spend our time gardening, walking in the woods, or floating down the river on large tubes. We're always cooking and we love to sing. On winter nights, we sit in front of the fire and talk into the early hours. People who visit Ravina agree that the conversations that happen there are magical. It was on one such wintry night that Murray and I were having a conversation. It started as an argument, but transformed into something else. We found ourselves communicating with an openness, and an ease that was surprising, as we were talking about some very painful and frightening aspects of our lives. We suddenly realised that this would be a conversation that would be worth sharing with an audience, not only the content of it, but the process of how it happened.

***Murray:*** We decided to take it on the road. We put in an abstract to present it at a family therapy conference in Montreal, which we did two years ago, for an audience of eight people. The audience reflections in Montreal took the story in a direction we could not have imagined, so we had to tell it again … and again and again. We have now told the story several times. Every time we tell it, we get to know one another more, and we find ourselves able to talk about things we could not previously have done. The telling of the story continues to be healing for us both.

Today we invite you to imagine yourselves at Ravina. The mountain, the forest and the river. Please join us for a chat in front of the fire.

***Paul:*** A month ago I re-visited my high school. It was the first time I had set foot on those grounds in twenty-one years. King David High School is a Jewish Day School in Johannesburg, South Africa. My time there was during the depths of the apartheid years, and all the children were white, and Jewish. A somewhat homogenous group, and if you didn't fit in, life was horrible. I spent my life at King David School afraid of the bullies who sat on the wall.

'Browde you queer. Come here pansy, rabbit, meet us on the top field for a battle, five o'clock we'll be there, bring your buddies.'

Thursdays were especially scary. Thursdays were known as rabbits' day, the days in which it was insinuated that boys did things with other boys. Certain boys were singled out as rabbits, and were teased relentlessly. I was never physically hurt by those boys, but they took up a lot of my energy. I became extremely vigilant at all times. While walking anywhere, if I noticed them out of the corner of my eye, I'd quickly change direction. I would walk for miles out of my way to avoid them as they sat there spitting words at everyone who passed them. If you got them one on one, they sometimes treated you okay.

I remember the relief I would feel when one of them was friendly ... the feeling that maybe it was over, maybe I was now accepted. But hours later, I'd see the same boy with his group of friends, and I knew in an instant that nothing had changed. I found a couple of the taller boys to spend my breaks with. As we stood and talked and ate our peanut butter sandwiches, I'd be scanning the area, alert, watching out for danger, ready for an attack.

I remember Murray from those days. He and I were in the same class and spoke to one another. I remember liking him. My first memory of him was at age thirteen. The teacher divided the class into pairs and told us to tell each other a story. Murray and I were partners in that exercise. But outside the classroom, Murray was someone I considered dangerous to be seen with. You see, it was all in Murray's body. He seemed weak to me. His shoulders were hunched, his neck bent forward. He never approached you head on, but always with his head slightly rotated to the side. There was a clumsiness to his hand movements. I could never imagine him fighting anyone. His body seemed to be saying 'don't notice me'. He was a weak boy with a pale body, and I hated that.

***Murray:*** Johannesburg. 1975. It was summertime. I was wearing my summer uniform. Long socks, khaki shorts and a matching safari jacket, with the school's emblem on its pocket: The Jewish star of David, the head of the Springbok (the animal that is South Africa's national symbol), and the open pages of a textbook. (These were the signs of my education. A Jew in South Africa.)

It was lunchtime. I had walked out of the classroom, forgetting my sandwiches, which my nanny Paula had packed for my lunch. Though the corridors were out of bounds during break times, I thought I'd make a quick dash for the classroom and retrieve my lunch. The classroom had big banks of windows facing the corridor. It was silent but for the distant voices on the playing field below.

I entered the classroom.

A voice shouted 'Look who we have here'.

And then there was laughter, loud laughter. I started towards the door. But they'd already surrounded me, blocking my exit. I knew all the boys, all the faces, all the names.

There was Myerson and Gavin and Joseph and Epstein.

They lifted my body and threw me down onto the wooden table at the front of the class. It smelled of chalk and lavender-scented wax. Their hands were all over me. Ten, twelve hands, punching, burning, pushing, twisting at my skin. And there were words. Pansy, sissy, morf. Pansy, pansy, pansy. Nossel you pansy, are you having a good time? I was silent. I didn't want them to hear me struggle. I tried to get up. Which made them thrust harder at limbs with their knuckles and their fists.

Look at him, thinking he can get away. And they lifted me towards the metal stationery closet. I knew what was next. I'd be put inside it, and then they'd turn the closet over and smash it against the wall. Then bash it with a cricket bat.

I managed to escape. I ran down the corridor, down the stairs out onto the stretch of lawn above the field. My arms and legs were branded with the deep red marks of their hands, which later turned to bruises.

***Paul***: Our Afrikaans teacher was completely unable to control the class. Most days she would storm out in tears. 'You kids are enough to make people anti-Semitic.' One particular day, and it was summer because we were wearing the beige safari suit summer uniforms, she decided to treat us like children and to punish us for being naughty. 'Okay class, if you are going to behave like kids I will treat you like kids.' She proceeded to herd us out of the classroom to the corridor outside. It was an upstairs classroom which looked down onto a grassy courtyard below.

'Now kids', she said in her quivering Afrikaans accent masquerading as tough, 'Boys on the right, and girls on the left'. There was a moment of silence, as I heard myself say 'and Murray in the middle'. Uproarious laughter erupted. Murray stood very still, I felt terrible, and I felt wonderful. I remember the relief. All eyes were focused on Murray. He was the object of derision. I was free. I was one of the guys and it felt great. It felt bad hurting this boy. I liked him, but I liked the relief more. The relief that I felt was worth any discomfort.

***Murray:*** It is Sunday afternoon in Johannesburg. I am listening to a record of Wagner's Valkyries. The bright sun forms a pool of light on the shelves of books which flank the wall. There is one book, a biography of Adolf Hitler. His face on its spine. A black image on a white background, and the words in red, Gothic print. Adolf Hitler. I lift out of my body, hovering above it looking directly at it. I see on my body the face of Adolf Hitler.

1976. It is quarter-to-nine on a Friday morning. The daily prayer service before school begins. I am among rows of boys. Our hands and heads are bound with the Tephilin, the leather straps of our Jewish faith. The religious boys are singing, swaying from side-to-side, deep in prayer. The prefects – with their distinctive blazers and badges – pace up and down the aisles, reprimanding boys for talking, chewing, laughing. Nonetheless there is a constant rumble of noise that isn't prayer or song. It is the sound of boys.

Ever since finding my seat, I have searched the room to locate my tormentors. Myerson, Epstein, Gavin, Joseph.

Myerson is standing in the next row. I drop my head immediately, but he catches me in my terror. It's too late to look away. He stings me with a sibilant 'sissy', mocking me with a limp wrist and a cocked head. He punches Epstein on the arm. I am encircled by their loud, derisive whispers. A prefect approaches. Myerson and Epstein fall silent. It's a moment of relief. I turn around, face the other way, look out of the window to the summer sky and the playing field. A punch stings my upper arm. I spin round. Myerson and Epstein are looking the other way, at the sea of girls in their blue pinafores. Who was it? Who punched me? I look at the boys surrounding me. It could be any one of them.

We are seated for the sermon. My head fills with Wagner's Valkyries. The orchestra surges and I begin to feel powerful, alive. I stand mighty, towering above Myerson and Epstein. Everyone, the boys, the girls, the prefects, the teachers look up towards me. Slowly, I peel my face away, to reveal underneath, the sculpted statue of a Nazi soldier. My eyes are no longer dark, but blue like the summer sky outside. I issue the command. My soldiers rise through the floorboards like spirits. Their uniforms are black, and their arms bear the insignia of the SS. I issue the command. Our flags are raised. Swastikas, eagles. Red, white, black, gold. Myerson and Epstein are the first to be led to the gallows, where they will be hanged in full view of everyone. The music is loud in my head, beautiful, triumphant.

Then suddenly something hits my neck. It is a piece of paper, rolled together with spit. The music stops abruptly. The statue crumbles. The soldiers disappear back into their spirit world.

The morning prayers are over. the teachers file onto the stage for the Friday morning assembly. A guest speaker has come to address the school. She is from New York, and her name is Esther Jungreis. She is a Rebbetzin, which means wife of a rabbi. She is tall, with blonde hair and a European accent. Her voice is strident. She tells us a story from her childhood. This is how I remember it. When Nazi soldiers arrived in her small Polish town, the Jews were rounded up, and taken to the town square. Her father, a rabbi, and all the other religious elders were led to the centre of the square. She watched as a soldier ripped her father's beard from his face, and shot a bullet through his head.

Her voice fills my head. All around me boys are biting their lips, trying not to cry. I am one of them. Ten miles away, soldiers are invading Soweto, the huge black township outside Johannesburg.

***Paul:*** 1981. Murray's body had changed. His hair was blond and long. His shoulders were more pulled back and his head was held high. He enunciated his words, wore black, and walked around the campus like an intellectual. Murray's body had changed and it was no longer weak. He had a group of intellectual artist friends. They smoked cigarettes and blew the smoke out forcefully as they laughed at the pathetic nerdy medical students of which I was one. I tried greeting Murray at times, but he would sweep past me with a brief, dismissing 'hi'.

***Murray:*** 1981. Kathy comes over to visit me and my boyfriend Ashley. She is furious and has come to us seeking comfort. She tells us she wants to have a relationship with a man, but he's gay. I press her for details. Finally she tells me, it's Paul Browde. I am more than pleased. It is a victory. It is thrilling news. I am excited. Paul Browde is on my team.

***Paul:*** 1984. San Francisco. I met Gary. I was 23 years old. Gary told me he was a social worker in an AIDS ward at a San Francisco Hospital. I was a medical student doing my elective in psychiatry up the hill. I was very interested in seeing what Gary did at work. I was also interested in an opportunity to feel a connection with one of these men. The gay clones of San Francisco. I had to remind myself that these men were gay, they were not the bullies from the wall at school.

I went to the ward and met the people who worked there. It was interesting and also shockingly sad. Young men were hooked up to IVs in the waiting room, watching re-runs of 'I love Lucy', chatting and laughing. These patients seemed used to their illness, they related to one another with humour and familiarity. All of them were young men with AIDS. Some were covered with the red spots of Kaposi Sarcoma, and all were very thin. Gary introduced me to the doctor in charge of the ward. One of the nurses showed me the whole set-up. I remember wishing that I worked in such a place, so gay-friendly, a place where people felt they belonged. Gary did great work, helping these men with services and counselling them. 'Whew, this is tough work', I thought. I was so struck by the contrast between Gary at work, doing service for his community, and Gary as one of the glazed-eyed, beer-drinking, pot-smoking, sex-talking men in Bobby's apartment where I'd met him. After work, Gary invited me to a party the following Saturday night. It was a birthday party of his upstairs neighbour, a well-known theatre person, in a very fancy area of San Francisco.

Saturday evening, I took time to get ready, dressing carefully, making sure I was well-showered and shaved. I dotted a little cologne on strategic points all over my body, including the little groove above my top lip, so that I could smell it. I entered the party a little daunted by the formality of it all, the tuxedos, the well-built, elegant men in white suits who harmonised with the women in black evening dress, as they milled around the white baby-grand piano. I chatted with a few people, and was of interest to some. I was an exotic foreigner, a medical student and a South African. I was tall, had dark curly hair, black eyes with thick jet-black eyebrows, and a persistent smile.

Gary arrived late. He was a slight man of average height. He had wavy brown hair, a narrow moustache, and a very childlike and open face. He was dressed in a checked flannel shirt with denim jeans, and seemed preoccupied and not particularly friendly. I was disappointed. I spent most of the evening eating snacks and listening to the classical pianist, who entertained to much applause. It was getting late and I decided to leave, said goodbye to Gary, and made my way down the steps to the street.

'Paul' – it was Gary calling out to me – 'Want to come in for a drink?'

I spun round with relief.

We entered his basement studio which was magically illuminated with tens of recently-lit candles. They cast a gentle light. He must have sneaked out of the party to prepare the room. There was tranquil music playing, creating a peaceful and romantic atmosphere, and Gary was charming, and beguiling. We had a passionate evening. The next day, I was in love. I knew where I could bump into Gary, and orchestrated doing so as soon as I could. The moment I saw him, I knew that Gary was clearly no longer interested. He was aloof and cold, and I was miserable and lonely.

The next day a friend of his called me and asked to meet with me. She told me over lunch that Gary was in a bad way, that the previous week he had found out that his T cells were abnormal. She told me that this meant that his immune system was damaged, that he was infected with the virus.

How could he be infected? I was baffled. He is a social worker, he would have told me, surely?

I had had unsafe sex with a man who was infected with HIV. What was going on in my mind? What was going to happen, and what was I to do?

***Murray:*** 1986. Cape Town. I began to have attacks of rigours. The experience of intense chills and trembling followed by profuse sweating. I consulted Dr G, a physician who had his offices in the medical centre where I was also practising as a psychologist at the time. He told me I had flu, prescribed Aspirin and sent me on my way. A week later, I collapsed during a consultation with a patient. My receptionist immediately helped me to Dr G's office. I was shaking uncontrollably and barely able to speak. Dr G asked if I'd ever had sex with men. I knew what he was thinking. 'It's impossible', I said, 'I can't possibly have AIDS'.

Nevertheless, he insisted that I be admitted to the hospital for tests. He didn't know what else to make of my symptoms. I asked if it couldn't be Malaria since I'd recently visited Central Africa. He rejected this explanation on the basis that I had taken my anti-malarial medication. 'No', he said, 'It is most likely AIDS'. The term AIDS had no meaning for me, except that the very sound of the word filled me with terror. All I knew was that it was a deadly disease that afflicted promiscuous homosexual men. On route to the hospital – in an already delirious state – I was visited by paranoid thoughts which seemed to go round and round in my mind. Had somebody deliberately pricked me with an infected needle? Was somebody trying to kill me? Did my lover have AIDS? I was admitted to an intensive care unit of Cape Town's General Hospital. Bloods were taken from me. They didn't give me sedatives. Racked with pain in my head and limbs, I lay awake the entire night, tortured by questions about what was happening inside my body. In the beds surrounding mine, men coughed incessantly throughout the night. The following morning I learned that I was in the tuberculosis ward. Shortly after sunrise, a cheerful medical intern informed me that I had tested positive ... for Malaria. In my relief, I forgot all about AIDS.

***Paul:*** 1985. I had noticed lumps behind my head. I felt them on the bony prominence behind my ear. I used to try and massage them away, to press them flat against my head. Soon there were more lumps, in my groin, under my arms, behind my elbows. I was in my final year of medical school, and try as I might to ignore them, after a while I had to take notice of them. My mother, an oncologist, was nonchalant about it. 'It's probably not serious. Let's put you on antibiotics and we'll see in six weeks.' Six weeks later there had been no change. 'Why don't we call Jack and ask him to biopsy one of them', my mother suggested. Jack was the father of one of my closest friends, and the best surgeon in town.

So it was that I took my lumps to Jack's office, where he recommended that I have the lymph node in my left armpit removed. Within days, a nurse was shaving my armpit smooth, and I was lying on the table, with my hand behind my head, Jack's warm eyes smiling above his green mask as he swabbed me with cold iodine. 'Count backwards from 10 to 1.' I woke up with stitches and a short stabbing pain under my left arm.

Five days later my mother got the results of the biopsy: 'non-specific inflammation'.

She was elated. 'I can tell you now. I have been so worried, you know me, I thought it was lymphoma.'

My family celebrated. My father popped champagne and toasted me: 'To good health, this is marvellous'. They all laughed with relief. I on the other hand did not feel relief. I knew. I knew that this was not the end. It was a vague, inchoate knowing. It was an unconscious horrified knowing, a dread, that I couldn't even speak to myself.

Some days later, Jack called me. He asked me to come and see him in his house, which I knew so well. I drove, more slowly than usual, up the winding road to the house. I walked into his study, and now, as if for the first time, I noticed the bookshelves, the desk, the leather chairs. It was early evening and the desk lamp cast a large shadow of Jack, who sat across from me, onto the beige curtains behind him. Jack's eyes were still friendly, but his face looked different. I was aware of his glasses perched on the bridge of his nose, his grey curls, and his large white teeth which seemed to grow as they began to move up and down in unison with his deep voice. He had begun to speak. 'Paul it is no secret that you are gay, everybody knows that.'

I was silent.

'So when you had the lymphadenopathy, I decided to test you for HIV, and I have to tell you, the results have come back positive.'

At that moment time began to play with me. The space between his revelation and my answer remains the longest moment I have ever lived. As if in trance, I experienced my life, and encountered my own death.

***Murray:*** The 20th June 1986. (I remember the day well. It was my twenty-fifth birthday.) I was contacted by Dr G, who asked whether I was willing to make a house visit to one of his patients who most urgently required psychological treatment. Why can't he come to my office? The physician was awkward. 'Well, he's recently become blind', he told me. Then added – with some trepidation – that the patient had AIDS.

My response was immediate. No. Absolutely not. I wouldn't do it. I was shocked, disturbed. Why was I hearing this word AIDS again? Why on my birthday? To confront a man, who (as Dr G put it) was having to come to terms with death. What about contagion?

Dr G assured me that one could not contract the disease casually. Specialists in America had come to this conclusion. Eventually I gave in. I felt it was my professional duty to go. I was told that the patient was residing in a building of holiday apartments, and that his diagnosis was strictly secret. If anyone found out he had AIDS, he'd be evicted immediately. I also learned that all hospitals in Cape Town, had rejected him. He was too contagious.

I parked my car outside the building – which was situated on a quiet street facing the Atlantic oceanfront – terrified of what I was going to discover. Terrified by my first-ever contact with AIDS, a disease that the Cape Town Press was calling the gay plague. Armed only with the hope that the 'American specialists were correct', and that I was not in any personal danger, I made my way to the room where my patient was (to put it plainly) being hidden. I rang the doorbell. I heard him stumbling. He extended his hand to greet me. I took a step backwards, avoiding his hand. He obviously sensed this. I went inside. The room was sad, chaotic. He was a gaunt man, unshaven and pale. His face was covered by dark purple spots. I noted that he coughed occasionally; and I made certain to sit what I considered a 'safe' distance away from him. I didn't know where to begin. What to say. What to ask him. Should I mention his illness? Should I ask him about death? I cannot remember what I asked him. I only remember that he began to cry, as he spoke to me in broken, barely comprehensible sentences. He battled to find words.

***Paul:*** I felt my voice rising, from my belly, up into my throat and out into the air which had become viscous, thick, holding the sound like smog, it echoed. 'Jack', I said, 'I wish you hadn't done that'.

'I didn't know whether to tell you or not. It has been a very difficult decision. I spoke to your GP, and we have agonised about whether or not to tell you. Your GP even called the Lubavitcher Rabbi in New York, and he thought we should tell you. We all agreed that I had to tell you.'

***Murray:*** I left the apartment and drove directly to my home, where I washed my hands, keys and pen in a powerful antiseptic. I had entered the plague, with its imagery of calamity, scourge and death. It was like a bad dream.

Dr G managed to have our patient admitted to a local psychiatric hospital, arguing that the patient had depression related to organic brain damage. About two weeks later, my patient died.

***Paul:*** The next few days were very slow. Nobody knew much about this condition. I consulted with a leprosy specialist who advised me to tell my mother the news. 'Look', he said, 'While we do our best to keep confidentiality, you never know. Your mother works in this system, and it's better she finds out from you than through the grapevine.'

I was sent to Dr B, a renowned and feared chemotherapist. He was an imperious man, who never looked me in the eye, but stared at his desk with no expression on his face as he listened to my story.

'Well, we need to do a battery of tests. You should have a whole lot of blood work done, and you need a bone marrow biopsy. Go into the next room and get undressed. I will do the bone marrow now.'

'Now?' I was terrified. I was well. I didn't feel sick. I had not prepared for this. I was not ready for this sudden assault on my body, being pricked and prodded everywhere. Dr B continued speaking to his desk: 'It has to be done, we may as well get it over with.' Within minutes he had pierced my hip with a wide-bored needle, plunging it deep into my bone marrow. 'You will feel some pressure as I pull back on the syringe', he warned me. Pressure was right. He failed to mention excruciating pain. I never got the results of the bone marrow biopsy, which I presume were negative.

It was around that time that my emotions switched themselves off. My life was bathed in a deadening numbness, which allowed me to complete my medical training. Troubled by the faint thought that I wasn't going to be around for very much longer, I decided shortly after completing my medical training to give up medicine completely and pursue my life-long dream of a career as an actor. I was accepted to start a full-time drama program the following August. All I needed was to live long enough to get there.

***Murray:*** 1990. I left South Africa. I wanted to pursue my life-long dream of a life as a playwright. By this time the so-called 'gay plague' had spread into the black townships and was reportedly being transmitted through heterosexual contact. But AIDS was no longer an issue in my life. I had been in a long-term monogamous relationship with a man; and, as far as I was aware, none of my friends were infected. Upon my departure from South Africa, concerned friends implored me to 'be careful' in New York, where the 'epidemic' was thought to be 'out of control'. I felt the reverberations of their warnings on the streets of Greenwich Village where the shadows of wasted bodies appeared and disappeared. Evidence of AIDS was everywhere. In the newspaper, on billboards, in the subways. Advertisements for condoms and safe sex were ubiquitous. I was determined to be careful; to keep AIDS out of my life.

Shortly after arriving in New York, I wrote my first play. It was called 'No Boundaries'.

A successful young French Canadian was recommended to me to be the director. It turned out that he was the lover of the man who told me to stand in the middle, Paul Browde.

In the course of the play's production, Paul and I began to have conversations.

***Paul***: I remember that I couldn't really feel comfortable with Murray until I had apologised. I wondered whether he remembered the sentence I had spoken fifteen years before.

***Murray:*** It was a sentence. I remembered it, and hearing the apology was a liberation. It was the beginning of my ability to extricate myself from a profoundly confusing past. It was the first time that the past had come back to greet me in a friendly way.

Within a few months, we were speaking to one another on a daily basis, oftentimes lamenting the fact that we had never previously developed a closer relationship.

***Paul***: I made it to drama school. It was a great experience, but acting as a career was not for me. But, it was at drama school that I met my partner, Simon, the French Canadian actor whose first gig in New York City was to direct Murray's play. Our relationship continues to be a wonderful, and exciting journey, but that's another story!!

After drama school I decided to do a residency in psychiatry.

It was in my third year that I had my first experience of conducting psychotherapy. The young man I was therapist to was in his early twenties and a medical student in a nearby hospital. One day, and out of nowhere, he came into the session with the question: 'How are your T cells?' I was completely stunned, unable to think, consumed with fear. I said: 'What are you talking about?'

'Your T cells. I know you are HIV positive, I saw it on the computer at the hospital.'

The hospital where he worked was also the hospital where I received my care.

'That is not true', I answered, 'You must have the wrong person'.

'Isn't your middle name Eric?' he asked.

I was cornered. I didn't know what to do. I held onto my seat till the session was over, and then froze in a rush of terror. He knew this thing about me that no-one at work knew. I was going to lose everything. My job, my career, my future. They were all over.

I didn't know who to turn to. It was a secret. I decided to take the risky step of telling my supervisor the truth about what was going on. Her response was 'love him, just keep loving him'. Given the way I was feeling, this was easier said than done. My therapist was helpful in getting me through the anxiety of that time. What was never addressed was the politics of secrecy. The fact that I belonged to a discriminated-against group. That I was forced to be silent. It was a couple of months later I realised that, until this was no longer a secret, I would never be free.

At that time, Murray was running a story-telling group at an AIDS day treatment program in Brooklyn. He encouraged me to come out as HIV positive. I trusted him. He said that, knowing me as he did, he was confident that this was a path to freedom.

***Murray:*** I encouraged Paul to speak out. I'd known a man who had died in silence, as a result of which, my community had been robbed of the value of his life, and the impact of AIDS on it. I was working with people at an AIDS day program and on a daily basis was experiencing the value of their stories. At first they thought they didn't have stories to tell, but as we grew together to recognise the power of listening, stories began to emerge. Some of the people I worked with made a decision to tell their stories publicly, and participating in the making of a video (Nossel 1999).

***Paul:*** I got together with a colleague whom I had met at an HIV positive doctors' support group, and together we designed a strategy. And so in Washington DC at the Annual Convention of the American Psychiatric Association, I revealed my long-held secret to a room of about fifty colleagues. I told the story of the young man who had discovered the truth about me. I spoke of how I had heard doctors speak of people living with HIV, and of how it affected me when I heard such comments as 'he's a goner'.

I spoke of how everything I had ever seen at the APA regarding HIV related to death, depression and dementia. I related to none of those categories. I spoke of how I had a happy life, and that my partner and my families of origin and of choice were supportive and loving. Living with HIV had transformed my life and their lives, in many and varied ways, and I was tired of hearing the subject whispered about in the hallways. There was a difference between privacy and secrecy.

I was free to tell or not to tell and no-one could use it against me again. My secret was no longer a secret.

## Reflections

***Murray:*** Our work together has shown us how there really is no separation between work and life. It continues to teach us how friendships and relationships are healing. Preparing this talk has been a process of retelling, remembering, healing, forgiving and apologising. In the past we have prepared for talks such as this one, and have had to deal with a certain amount of conflict regarding the ownership of stories. I often felt that I was there to provide a background for Paul's story, and because I was HIV negative, was not entitled to tell my own story. I resented Paul for reminding me that I was HIV negative at times. At the same time, I felt that the HIV positive identity was so much mine, especially given the fact that my life partner has an HIV diagnosis. As such, it is my story.

***Paul:*** For me it was difficult to accept that Murray's experience of HIV was the same as mine. We found ourselves struggling to create a unified experience, at the same time each yearning to voice our separate identities. I had something in my body that Murray didn't have. I had to take medication five times a day and he did not. I had physical side-effects of these medications and he didn't.

HIV is an integral part of who I am. I recognise that it will live with me for the rest of my life. I can hate it, or I can learn to love it. I find myself reacting when people talk about wiping out the virus – it's my body they are referring to. HIV has taught me so much, about what's important in life, about forgiveness, about love. As such, it is my story.

***Murray:*** I came to realise that I am HIV negative. I do not take medication. I do not have side-effects, and I consciously practise safe sex in order to avoid becoming infected. HIV negative in the context of this discussion has become a conscious identity. I choose to remain HIV negative.

***Paul:*** In preparing for this talk we found ourselves struggling less for ownership of the story. Murray described feeling completely included in the process, rather than just a provider of context for me. I found myself trusting him in a way I hadn't before. I believe his acknowledgement that we are different, that his experience is not mine, has relieved me. I find myself able to listen to his experience with compassion. We are conscious of the struggle for ownership of the story, and continue to give up that struggle on an ongoing basis. Two weeks ago, in preparation for this conference, we spent forty-eight hours unearthing memories, retelling stories that we have told one another countless times. Finding inside them new meanings, new feelings. We looked at our old school photographs searching for the monsters we had been describing in our recollections. We were shocked and almost disappointed to find only the faces of gangly adolescents posing awkwardly for the group photographs. We found ourselves crying and laughing and discovering in our relationship a new level of intimacy, which involved talking about things that we had been too afraid to talk about before. We spoke about our reactions and thoughts about one another's bodies, a conversation we had never had before. We came to realise that there are still some stories that we do not feel comfortable or ready to tell in a public setting.

***Murray:*** Ultimately this talk is not about either one of us. We have used our experiences and our stories as a way of understanding how people hurt one another, how they find compassion, and how they forgive. I was worried about how my life would sound to people in this audience, especially other Jews. A Jewish boy fantasising himself into the body of a Nazi. This was an extreme measure and I cannot apologise for the fact that it happened, but I can forgive myself knowing that it has been my life- long endeavour to understand why that happened to me in the face of my own terror.

I forgive the victimised silent boy at school. I forgive myself for finding refuge in images of Nazi Germany.

I forgive Myerson. I forgive Epstein.

I forgive Joseph. I forgive Gavin.

I forgive the doctor who mis-diagnosed me. I forgive myself for letting a man die in silence. I forgive Paul.

***Paul****:* I forgive myself for humiliating Murray. I forgive myself for being frightened. I forgive my doctor for taking my blood while I was asleep.

I forgive Gary. I forgive HIV.

# PART FOUR

# *Therapy and lesbian lives*

In this section, Claire Ralfs and Manja Visschedijk explore the politics of therapy and how this relates to lesbian experience.

# 15

# A reflection on 'couple therapy'

by

Claire Ralfs

I am not a therapist and so this short reflection is written from my experiences of couple therapy (much of which has been pretty difficult and some an out right disaster), my conversations with other lesbians, and my engagement with narrative practices. In this piece of writing I have tried to convey some aspects of what I believe is often problematic for lesbians (and others) when they enter the therapy room and to provide some ideas towards an alternative framework to 'couple therapy'.

**From 'the couple' to 'partnerships'**

First of all, it seems that in much of the work of 'couple therapists' there is a complete absence of a critique in relation to the assumptions that people *should* couple and that the performance of coupledom should be central in our lives. Within western culture, there is a strong heterosexual dominant, nuclear family template that privileges relationships between couples. This privileging of one sort of relationship over all others is often significantly problematic. Clearly, it is problematic for other relationships people may have such as with their children, friends, colleagues, parents and extended families. It is also often problematic for the couple relationship itself. When the couple relationship fails to provide the (unrealistic) rewards expected of it, then the relationship itself, rather than the assumptions of coupledom, is often harshly judged.

An alternative to privileging the relationship of the couple is to privilege instead a metaphor of partnership. If therapists orientated to the question 'What could this partnership be/do/offer' this may create a range of different options outside the discourse of coupledom. When two people then enter a therapy room, perhaps some starting points could be:

- What has held your partnership together even though you have different histories, interests?
- What are some of the purposes/hopes of this partnership?
- What does this relationship mean to you in your individual and shared lives?
- What is the history of the idea of wanting to improve your relationship?
- How are these ideas operating?

These sorts of questions might assist the therapeutic conversations to move away from the format of 'working on person A's issues' and then 'working on person B's issues' and instead create a context for conversations about people's shared and separate hopes and dreams, the histories of these, and the particular practices that may contribute to moving towards them. Process of definitional ceremony could be used in this process, whereby one member of the couple is interviewed while the other acts as an outsider witness.

Being able to develop discursive resources that allow both people to discuss a negotiated and shared idea of the relationship, including its purposes, hopes and what it stands for in their separate and shared lives would seem to me to be a useful place to begin a therapy process. I believe that if these conversations were to take place, then rich descriptions of the hopes and purposes of relationship could be articulated.

## Explicitly externalising the broader discourses of relationships

I also wonder if a conversation about the broader ideas about 'couple relationships' might be useful for some people when they enter therapy together. The nuclear family paradigm remains so dominant that the specific hopes and dreams of individuals and couples are all too often obscured. At the same time, the assumed practices of couple life – shared bank accounts, sexual monogamy, living together and giving up most of our other friendships and relationships except those of our shared children – are notoriously difficult. The prescriptions about couple relationships are so pervasive that explicitly discussing these broader influences might free people up to more easily identify their own preferences for the shape of their relationship, the places where they have gotten off track and possible steps for the future.

## From privatising couple-life to locating the relationship in community

A further complicating factor is the way in which the discourse of coupledom shapes how the details of couple's relationships remain private. This privatising of couple life seems to me to be a mechanism that isolates couples from their other relationships. Finding ways for the 'partnership' relationship to be situated within a community of relationships, I believe, makes it possible for the couple involved to negotiate more satisfactory ways of relating. Being able to engage in a variety of relationships with different people in ways that are valued can take considerable pressure off the couple.

Therefore, in 'couple therapy' when other relationships are mentioned in the conversations, perhaps it can be identified if these other relationships contribute to the shared purposes of the partnership:

- Are there ways in which these friendships support the partnership?
- If so, how could the particular practices of support be further engaged with / responded to?
- If not, are there other relationships that you consider support the partnership, and how?

- How could the particular practices of support be further engaged with / responded to?

Locating the partnership in this broader community context may also make the task of recognising and responding to class, cultural and gender differences between partners less hazardous. Discursive resources that allow the individuals to think about and discuss these issues in broader terms than the specifics of their individual actions and relationships may become more available and this seems important.

**Summary**

In this short piece I've tried to convey some of the pitfalls that I believe are associated with much 'couple work'. These include a lack of a critique of the dominant discourses of coupledom, and a lack of awareness of the privatisation of intimate relationships. I have tried to briefly offer an alternative conception of working with the metaphor of partnership, of explicitly discussing the broader discourses of couples, and of being attentive to locating the partnership within a broader community of relationships.

Within these considerations, it becomes possible to envisage ways of working that rather than aiming to help couples work towards fitting in with the 'romantic bliss/sexual fidelity/economic security' discourses that so dominate our culture's understanding of what a couple relationship should look like, instead create space for people to articulate and move towards their preferred ways of relating.

Perhaps the therapy room could become a place where, instead of further validating the dominant discourses about couples, the unconventionality and particularity of many people's partnerships could be honoured, explored and more richly described. I believe this would make the therapy room a more relevant and inviting place not only for lesbians, but for anyone whose ideas of relationship do not fit the nuclear family template.

# 16

# A reflection on Changing Our Minds: Lesbian feminism and psychology

*co-authored by*
*Celia Kitzinger & Rachel Perkins*
*(1993, New York University)*

by

Manja Visschedijk

**Introduction**

> *Psychological diagnoses are taking the place of political debate ...* [and] *has replaced feminism as a way of understanding the world.* (Kitzinger & Perkins 1993, p.6)

Although I don't completely agree with it, I like this bold statement, for much the same reason as I like this book, *Changing Our Minds*, for the robustness of its argument.

How did 'the personal is the political' become the 'personalising' of the political? This question, which is a key theme of the book, is, to my mind, as intriguing and relevant to discussions about 'the politics of therapy' today as it was nine years ago, when this book was published. I found myself wondering whether the authors too, still found their arguments relevant and if and where they might have shifted position? It is my hope that my reflections and your reading of them will contribute to the continuing co-construction of this important body of knowledge, which I would call the 'politics of therapy'.

For those of you who haven't read the book, it turns a critical eye upon the lesbian feminist community to which the authors belong, revealing a disturbing predilection for psychological accounts of lesbian lives, relationships and community. Lesbian feminists, the authors argue, have embraced the promotion of psychological interpretations wholeheartedly and blindly – with problematic consequences. Since the dominant culture – the wider English speaking Western culture – uses psychology to promote its values and ethics (including heterosexual dominance), then the use of psychology by lesbian feminists to interpret experience must necessarily incorporate those values and ethics. As well as exposing ourselves blindly to a value system frequently at odds with our own, the authors argue, we also contribute to the construction of a world in which the individual is paramount; political concerns are translated into private ones; social change depends on a 'revolution from within', and success is determined by how an individual feels, and this can only be detrimental to a marginalised community.

In challenging the prevalence of psychology, the authors advocate for a revival of ethical and political debate and action in every arena of lesbian life, ousting psychology from its place as chief organiser of our thinking and as key tool for the shaping of our aspirations for action. The way forward, they argue, is to ditch psychology altogether, because, in their view, it is fundamentally incompatible with lesbian feminist politics and undermining of lesbian feminist community.

In the reading of this book I experienced new insights resulting from both the 'yes!' of resonances with my own thoughts, dilemmas and conclusions and the happy friction arising at those places where I felt compelled to part company with the authors central arguments and move into the less polarised territories of what I understand by 'the politics of therapy', territories in which feminism and 'therapeutic' work can act as partners in ways which progress the projects of both.

My reflections as I read included the following 'yes':

- the invasion of psychological language into lesbian communities and the role this language plays in usurping political analysis and debate.
- the implications of psychology's translation of 'ordinary feelings and painful reactions to the vicissitudes of life' into 'poor mental health' (Kitzinger & Perkins 1993, p.74).
- the pathologising of lesbian relationships, for example in the use of such terms as 'internalised homophobia' and 'merged relationships'.
- the organisation of lesbian identity around the ways in which we have been wounded.

... and the following points of departure:

- a movement away from polarising the issue in ways that close down possibilities, such as saying 'feminism is incompatible with psychology'.
- an interest in exploring the multiple manifestations of both feminism and psychology, to see if options for feminist practice within the realms of the psychologies arise.
- a proposition for devising alternative metaphors, other than that of 'wounding', 'damage' or 'victimhood', around which to organise identity, such as 'belonging', or the 'knowing formation of identity'.
- thinking about the kinds of therapeutic spaces that might be needed to enable the active participation of people and communities in the knowing formation of identities.

If I were still primarily influenced by academic practices I might now proceed to elaborate on these points in an orderly fashion, however since I prefer to write in ways shaped by quilt-making practices, I will allow my reflections to emerge patchwork-wise, while hopefully keeping the authors and their book respectfully at the centre of my writing, and you (dear reader), with some sense of the pieces making a pleasing, but open-ended whole.

As a lesbian feminist currently working as a manager in a mainstream relationship counselling agency, with a history of working as a counsellor within the youth and women's sector, and with an abiding interest in examining my own work in relation to the politics of therapy, I feel I have something to say on this subject and I intend to engage with the above points in a spirit of passionately honing our politics and our ethics, by '… disagreeing with each other, challenging and criticising each other's perspectives' (Kitzinger & Perkins, 1993, p.151), which the authors argue is critical to the building of a viable lesbian community, a sentiment with which I fully agree.

In this spirit also, I want to flag a further abiding dilemma about my speaking position in this conversation when I use the words 'we' and 'our'. Although I have lived, loved and worked for 24 years as a part of this feisty, inspiring, challenging, rewarding and delightful community, it is not the only community to which I belong. As a mother to a son, aunt to nephews, sister to brothers, daughter to a father, friend to heterosexuals and sometimes lover to male partners, I have not been comfortable when my lesbian feminist community, by its very naming, is closed to these beloveds and hence divides me from them.

While I have understood the historical need for naming and claiming lesbian feminist discursive and geographical space, have joined the struggle to win this space, and have accommodated the resulting dilemmas in various more or less successful ways, they have never been satisfactorily resolved, and while I am not going to talk about these things in this article, I do want to acknowledge how the work of Esben Esther Pirelli Benestad and Elsa Almaas, (Benestad 2001) has opened new pathways for me with regard to identity issues. By arguing convincingly, as they do, that there are in fact more than two expressions of gender, they offer me a way to imagine more than two expressions of sexual identity – not an expression of 'bi-sexual identity, as this again presumes and confirms two possible expressions of sexuality – but something else, some perhaps more fluid and dynamic expression of sexuality, which, if I knew what it was, I would name my speaking position as!

My reflections then, are as a 'lesbian in search of a third expression of sexuality' and as a feminist practitioner of 'therapy', working with people belonging to a diversity of communities, and bringing a range of issues and concerns to the therapeutic consultations.

**Feminism and psychology?**

Returning then to the authors' central argument, that feminism is fundamentally incompatible with psychology (Kitzinger & Perkins 1993, p.6). Maybe its the influence of my current workplace, but I don't believe that these two should 'divorce' so much as re-negotiate the terms of their relationship, and subject this relationship to a continual reflexive process, framed by a thorough articulation of feminist ethics and politics. They could, for example, ask of the relationship, 'how much are you being influenced by the ideas and practices of heterosexual dominance?'; 'how do you know this?'; 'are there any occasions when this is not so?'; 'which ideas and practices would you prefer the relationship to be influenced by?' and 'what do you know about elevating those preferred ways?'. They could ask of the relationship, 'how much are you being influenced by the primacy of ideas about 'coupleness', duality and polarities?'

One of the first and most significant places at which I parted company with the authors was in their use of the strategy of polarising the issue, using the polarity as a frame to hold the main threads of their unfolding argument. While I agree with the authors that there are times to make moral and ethical stands, and to argue strongly for a particular political position at a given point in time, I think that the statement: 'feminism and psychology are incompatible' erodes any uses it may have had in marking a line at which to make a political stand by contributing to the creation of absolute positions and by closing down options for people to take action on their own behalf. Anyway, which psychologies and which feminisms are they talking about?

In my view, binaries and polarities are the especial friends of hetero-patriarchy, and are key players in the marginalisation of some communities. In polarising black and white; homosexual and heterosexual; female and male, the discourses of white-hetero-patriarchy are strengthened. In which case it could be argued that the authors are reproducing precisely that which they set out to dismantle. I wonder what they would say to this, nine years on from the time at which they wrote?

Rather than polarise the issue in this way, I would have preferred the authors to turn their wonderful deconstructive abilities – as evidenced in their insightful spotlighting of psychology's tricks throughout their book – upon the politics of particular therapeutic practices.

Questions I would have liked them to turn their eagle gaze upon include:

- What are the effects of 'professionalising practices' on therapeutic practices- when the voices of academics and therapists are privileged above the 'insider knowledges' of those who have lived particular experiences?
- What are the effects of the structures in which therapies are practiced? What does it mean to go into a small room with a 'professional' and expose your most painful memories? What difference does it make to talk about these things with a small group of others who have travelled similar paths? or to talk about these things around a kitchen table or out under trees or in a pool hall?
- Does it matter where we practice therapies? how bodies are arranged in space and who speaks first?

Again, I wonder what the authors might have to say about some of the feminist thinking that has developed around these themes. For instance, I'd like to get their opinion of Alcoff & Gray's proposition that: 'Speech is an event involving the arrangement of speakers and hearers; it is an act in which relations get constituted and experience and subjectivities are mediated ... In many speaking situations some participants are accorded the authoritative status of interpreters and others are constructed as the "naive transmitters of raw experience"' (Alcoff & Gray 1993, p.264).

Or what they might have to say about Johnella Bird's observations that the 'conventional use of English supports the strong adherence to polarities such as success/failure, belongs/abandoned, forgiveness/resentment. These polarities function to categorise, measure and assess.' Instead of parting company with therapy however, Bird works to engage with it in ways which expose the political nature of both the structure and the meanings of words within the English language '... in moving away from these polarities ... we create opportunities to generate *language for the inbetween* (Bird 2000, pp.20-23).

I can't accept that we have to choose, either therapy or politics, and the authors did not convince me that the lesbian feminist community, or any other marginalised community would be better off for having done it. Anyway, how are they planning to sever the relationship? If psychology is so pervasive, then how can we hope to find a place outside of it? Surely our best way forward is to find the cracks in its seemingly unified and monolithic facade and between us find ways to harness its resources to our own purposes and intentions.

## The significance of language

Another way forward is in exposing psychology's tactics through deconstruction of its key terms and major claims, which is precisely what Alcoff & Gray's problematising of the acts of speaking and Bird's thoughts on the significance of linguistic practices achieve – so too, do Kitzinger and Perkins in their chapter on language, and the content of our everyday speech. 'Psychobabble', they say, 'is increasingly replacing political language'. (Kitzinger & Perkins 1993, p.33).

In their chapter called 'watching our language', they show how 'psychobabble' is a key agent of psychology's infiltration of our communities. Pointing to the proliferation of words like 'co-dependent'; 'twelve-step'; 'being in recovery' 'inner child', 'processing', 'personal growth', 'the revolution within' etc, they argue that the de-politicising of language carries serious implications for lesbian politics, lives and community, since language reflects and constitutes our political analysis.

I have to agree! We are what we speak! I have often used this kind of language and have heard it in the descriptions proferred by the people who consult me about their issues and concerns, as well as among the conversations of friends and colleagues. This linguistic invasion holds several possible hazards and the authors outline three of the different strategies psychology has used ' … to infiltrate our vocabulary. It has co-opted and redefined existing political words; it has invented new depoliticised terms of its own; and it has tried to ban words from our vocabulary' (Kitzinger & Perkins 1993, p.37).

Words like 'liberation', 'power', 'choice' and 'rights' have been co-opted to take on individualised and pathologised meanings. For example, a 'woman of power' in this co-opted version, indicates a woman in touch with her authentic, natural feminine self. Every woman, this psychologised account infers, already has this power within her, she just needs to 'find' or 'liberate' it. As the authors point out, a worrying consequence of this is that the idea of political power – the power to stop male violence, enable access to education, jobs, land, money – recedes to the far margins of the conversation, leaving a familiar woman-blaming idea in its place, since, if women have access to this inner power, then it can only be their own fault if they are poor, get assaulted or dumped by their husbands or lovers!

Another point, in relation to language, which I found interesting, was the authors observation that words, such as 'should' and 'ought', which, in their view, carry important moral meanings, speaking to lesbian values and ethics, and which can delineate our responsibilities and acceptable ways of behaving within our communities, have been casualties of psychology's campaign to replace political analysis in our lives. Psychologists, the authors argue, who advocate for us to do away with the 'tyranny of the shoulds', deprive us of constructing principled positions from which to act. Instead of asking ourselves the moral question, 'is this right or wrong?' we are encouraged by psychology to ask, 'is this going to work for me?' (Kitzinger & Perkins 1993, p.67). With words of moral significance shorn from our language, the authors point out, we lose the possibility of developing a collective sense of lesbian ethics and lesbian values. 'The result is psychology's colonisation of our political terrain' (Kitzinger & Perkins 1993, p.72).

I agree with their arguments but not necessarily with their conclusions. I don't like their use of the word 'colonisation' because I don't think you can compare the struggle over the meanings of the words 'should' and 'ought' with the stealing of whole languages, people's land and cultures and customs. I also believe that it is possible – vitally important! – to include a consideration of ethics in the everyday theorising and practice of therapy.

**The pathologising of the ordinary**

> *Once all lesbians were sick simply by virtue of being lesbian. Now, some lesbians are self-actualised and fulfilled while others are ... not necessarily 'sick', but functioning sub-optimally* (Kitzinger & Perkins 1993, p.93).

Psychology, the authors argue, has created a thriving business for itself in fostering the view that ordinary lesbians are unable to move through the break-up of a relationship, the hassles of 'coming out'; the frustrations of dealing with heterosexual families, or the dilemma's of sex and intimacy without professional, therapeutic assistance (Kitzinger & Perkins 1993, p.73). Yes! I thought to myself, and, how did this happen?

According to the authors, '... much of what goes on in therapy – witnessing another lesbian's pain, listening attentively to her story, acknowledging her struggles – can and should be part of the ordinary business of friendship' (Kitzinger & Perkins 1993, p.84).

Another important ethical point which caught my attention in the book was the fact that in the case of severe difficulties, when we could expect psychology, rather than everyday friends to step in, many therapists refuse to see these clients, sending them off on a round of referrals across different institutions, and in and out of several offices, often thereby increasing, rather than easing, the suffering of those people the authors have named as 'mad or 'socially disabled' lesbians (Kitzinger & Perkins 1993, p.153).

> *Few private therapists in the United Kingdom will even see someone who carries a label from the psychiatric system, and someone who is too distressed to hold down a job would be unlikely to be able to pay for psychotherapy in any case.* (Kitzinger & Perkins 1993, p.74)

In allowing this, they point out, we fail in our moral and ethical responsibilities as members of lesbian community. There are some things, the authors strongly assert, which we 'ought' to do, and caring for the 'disabled' members of our communities is one of them. Again, I have to agree, although I don't like the word 'disabled' at all – for several reasons, including the fact that it organises identity around a polarity and around a metaphor of wounding, damage, and victimhood.

**The wounded or fragile self**

The authors answer to the moral and ethical vacuum caused by the infiltration of psychobabble into our conversation, is to develop a political analysis of our 'miseries'. In some ways I agree! 'Ordinary feelings, painful reactions to the normal vicissitudes of life – despair, anger, grief, frustration – have now become "problems" in need of psychological treatment' (Kitzinger & Perkins 1993, p.74). I have heard this with my own ears! But I wonder if the authors have considered the fact that for some people the opposite is true? Mary Gilfus, in her article 'The price of the ticket', observes that: '... trauma research [often] includes only a limited measure of abuse to document the source of the trauma and a standardised symptom checklist to demonstrate the pathology associated with it' (Gilfus 1999, p.1242).

The political consequences of this are that some experiences get counted as legitimate trauma – car accidents, sexual violence etc, while others are discounted – day-to day racism, poverty, unemployment. There are clear race, gender and class biases operating in the construction of psychological theory, with the very real effects of increased suffering for some people, when the purported aim of psychology is to relieve it.

While the politics of misery and suffering may be more complex than the authors had initially considered, there still remains for me the question, how much do we want to theorise our misery anyway? Without actually asking this question, the authors do allude to some possible hazards of centring our misery. 'We are encouraged ... to organise our identities around our frailties, our inadequacies, our wounds' (Kitzinger & Perkins 1993, p.135).

If we did not organise therapy around problems, around damage, wounds and injuries, what would we be doing instead? Conversely, if the authors are correct in their observation that psychology has taken the place of political analysis, then what would be the effect of pressing therapy into the service of politics, in for example, the project of performing meaning around preferred identities? Is this what the members of the elderly Jewish community in Venice California demonstrated to Barbara Myerhoff when she researched their lives? The importance for people to be seen '... and in one's own terms, garnering witnesses to one's worth, vitality and being' (Myerhoff 1986, p.267).

I know that for myself, the experience of sewing a story quilt, over the course of an eighteen month period, in the company of family and friends, then taking it into the public forum of the 2001 Narrative Conference in Adelaide, had profound 'therapeutic' benefits for me, without ever needing to centre the 'wounding' caused by dominant culture accounts of our identity as an illegitimate, unhealthy, unsuccessful family (Visschedijk, 2001).

**Individualising practices**

How did 'the personal is the political' become the personalising of the political? As I said at the beginning of this article, I think this very important point is as relevant today as at the time of the authors' writing. Having worked as a counsellor with the effects of sexual assault on people's lives, I have had many encounters with psychology's habit of individualising problems! The authors bring a sense of humour as well as their skills of political analysis to their explanation of how psychology has gained such prominence on behalf of individualising practices.

According to psychology, the authors explain: 'each of us has a very special possession called a "self", and we are all responsible for discovering, affirming, loving and improving that "self"'. They point to a mountain of literature that takes up this theme of self-loving – a multitude of books with titles such as *Learning to love yourself*; and *Courage to be yourself*, or if you can't manage that yet, then *Accepting yourself* or *Reclaiming yourself* will have to do until you can attain *Living in love with yourself* (Kitzinger & Perkins 1993, p.108). All this loving and affirming is needed because these individual selves are also seen as 'fragile and needy' (Kitzinger & Perkins 1993, p.135).

While these excesses of psychology's elevation of the 'fragile, needy self', do lend themselves to the ridicule with which the authors serve them, I still don't think this is reason enough to abandon therapeutic books altogether. If the authors could read *Telling our stories in ways that make us stronger* by two Indigenous Australian women Barbara Wingard and Jane Lester (2001), they might see that individuals are not paramount in every community, just as in many languages there is no word equivalent to 'psychology' or 'therapy'. As the authors themselves point out: 'The concept of the private and innermost "self" to be discovered, affirmed and loved by each individual is a peculiarly Western notion' (Kitzinger & Perkins 1993, p.112).

I wonder if the authors have shifted at all, since 1993, in their conclusion that 'lesbian feminism', and 'psychology', are inherently incompatible? I wonder too, if they have given any more consideration to their brief acknowledgement of the implications of the effects of culture in relation to these issues. For myself, these considerations play an important part in my conviction that there *is* a way to accommodate both politics and the wellbeing of the mind.

**'Therapy' as social activism**

There are, I believe, many examples of therapies that incorporate a political analysis – would the authors dismiss all of these, or have these proliferated in the years since their book was published? I would like to ask them, if therapy is not organised around the concept of a single, individual self, but around the concept of a complex web of relationships then do you think the outcomes could be different?

The examples of therapies that are involving political analysis and social action are numerous and include the following:

- The Family Centre, from Lower Hutt in New Zealand (Tamasese & Waldegrave 1994, Tamasese, Waldegrave, Tuhaka & Campbell 1998) provide but one example of the compatibility of politics and a therapy that is grounded in processes and structures of accountability.
- In an article entitled 'Activism and Optimism' by Susie Costello, Sue Jackson and Luke Jackson (Costello, Jackson & Jackson 2001, pp.71-96), links are made between global politics and the concerns that people bring to therapy.
- In the field of drug and alcohol counselling, political and social action are intricately linked to the wellbeing of people and their communities: 'In the broader culture, drug use is seen in many ways. It is seen as a medical issue, a psychological issue, an issue of criminality, a social issue. What is missing here is that drug use is primarily and embarrassingly a political issue' (Moss & Butterworth 1999, p.96).
- The work of Michelle Cherubin, Wendy Flynn & Aerinn Morgan, as written up in their article: 'Towards power and change: working with women carers within the mental health system' (Cherubin, Flynn & Morgan 1998, pp.7-22), incorporates politics into therapeutic practice.
- The organisation Women and Mental Health describes themselves as 'a group of consumers, carers, workers, or providers of mental health services' who 'discuss issues (such as the links between homelessness, sexual violence, or cultural experience and mental health) and work for change' (WAMH flier 2002).
- Sisters Inside describe themselves as 'an independent community organisation which exists to advocate for the human rights of women in the

criminal justice system in Queensland and to address gaps in the services available to them' (Sisters Inside mission statement). On their website (www.sistersinside.com.au), Sisters Inside indicate that they work alongside women in prison in determining the best way to fulfil the counselling and community work roles they undertake.

I wonder what Celia Kitzinger and Rachel Perkins would say to a proposal for 'a coalition of consumers, carers, workers, or providers of services' with the understanding that these were not distinct categories but that any woman might cross from being provider to consumer to worker etc?

And I wonder what you, the reader, would say in response to all of this.

For myself, I look forward to carrying these conversations forward and continuing these discussions among my own friends and colleagues both within the lesbian feminist community and outside of it, in the tradition of bold statements and robust argument, of which the book, *Changing Our Minds* is such a fine example.

# PART FIVE

# *Therapeutic work with gay men*

What follows are two practice-based papers describing work with gay men. The first paper, by Christopher Behan, focuses on group work. The second, by Bill Logan, describes a narrative approach to telephone counselling. This paper is then followed by thoughtful reflections from a range of therapists.

# 17

# Linking lives around shared themes

## Narrative group therapy with gay men

by

Christopher Behan

This paper is an expression of my experience of leading a gay men's group for the past six years in my practice at the Family Institute of Maine in North America. As such, many of the ideas may pertain most relevantly to practice with gay men. However, I will attempt as well to offer some ideas about how what I have learned could be useful to any narrative therapist doing what has been traditionally known as group therapy. I believe there is a great deal more to be said about group work from a narrative perspective. It is my hope that others will continue to add to this body of knowledges, skills and practices.

What has emerged from my experience and my studies in narrative therapy is a conviction that the idea of definitional ceremony, as proposed by Barbara Myerhoff (1978) and expanded by Michael White (1995), is at the centre of this work. Both writers talk about how authenticity is the outcome of a social process where one's preferred identity claims are acknowledged. Through definitional ceremonies, peoples' stories are linked around shared beliefs, commitments and purposes. White (1995) has outlined how reflecting team methodology can be applied for this purpose of linking lives around shared themes. I would like to describe how the use of therapy groups as reflecting teams can contribute to the richer description of its members' lives. In these groups the reflecting team is made up of peers instead of psychotherapy professionals, as has been most common up until now. In this way, the therapy group becomes both a reflecting team and a community of concern (Madigan & Epston 1995).

Myerhoff describes how definitional ceremonies were *contrived to arouse great emotion and energy, which was then redirected toward some commonalities, some deep symbols, and shared stable norms* (1978, p.185). Indeed, she writes of how these collective dramas contribute to the construction of the 'self'. Here she describes a man who was writing his autobiography:

> *Through the heightened awareness and consciousness provided by self-reflection, he was crossing the delicate threshold between merely being and being a man, a sentient human being, knowing himself to be. In order to accomplish this one needs reflecting surfaces ... Audiences, listeners, witnesses are essential for self awareness.* (pp. 221-222)

Following these ideas, I wish to write about an approach to group work in which the communal aspects of therapy are emphasised. This type of community assists its members in making meaning of their identity by seeing themselves and the world through multiple lenses. Lynn Hoffman (1998) talks about the idea of therapy as a 'kind of collective social weaving, like the Bayeux tapestry' where 'natural assemblies of people' are called together to create 'a more richly nuanced picture' of those present (p.7). In this way, the common narrative of 'finding your own voice' is a communal achievement. I think there is a great potential in this idea of making use of natural assemblies of people in therapy, those who surround the person in life, family, friends or any community of concern. Using group members as reflecting teams is just one of an infinite number of possibilities. In the work described below, the group acts as outsider witnesses for gay men who have few forums where they can be acknowledged, since so many of them are cut off from their families or live in relative isolation.

I must add that for me the process of being a participant in these groups contributes richly to my own sense of who I am and who I want to be. I assume there will be real effects on me as a result of my interactions with the group members. I have been changed (and continue to be changed) by being with these fellows. As another gay person, I do not see these persons who consult me as other than who I am or as something exotic.

**Background**

When I first began running a group for gay men, I had a lot to unlearn. Fresh from graduate school my head was inculcated with ideas about what constituted good group practice and my role as expert. Structuralist ideas had informed my learning about group therapy. At the same time, I started my work with a fervent hope to mitigate the suffering that these gay men were feeling, which I had experienced myself. I quickly saw how many of the taken-for-granted practices of therapy in groups did not fit for the men with whom I was working. For example, I knew that there were problems with the sacrosanct idea that group members could not have contact with each other outside of the group meetings.

It seemed cruel to me to introduce gay men to each other, many of whom were newly claiming their sexual identities and extremely isolated socially, and then forbid them to have contact. So, as I began the group, I knew I had to let the group members get to know each other outside of the group context. The idea that I had been taught of the group as an isolated social microcosm used to create a 'corrective emotional experience' (Yalom 1985, p.19), had to go out the window. In order to be more helpful to the men in the group, I had to find other ways to conceive of this undertaking.

Over time, the group has evolved with my growing knowledge of narrative therapy, through trial and lots of error, and from feedback from the group members. I wanted to create a context where people could find an audience to witness the stories of their lives. Rather than a group effort which continues to enshrine the individual, contributing to more isolation and loneliness, I wished to participate in group work which would act as a forum in which people's stories could be linked around shared beliefs and shared commitments. Eliciting and linking stories has become a key aspect of the group. I have been influenced by Sharon Welch's understandings of this:

> *The function of telling particular stories of oppression and resistance is not to find the 'one true story' of subjugation and revolt but is to elicit other stories of suffering and courage, of defeat, of tragedy and resilient creativity.* (1990, p.139)

For most of the history of this group, we followed what I would call a fairly common group therapy format. There was an unstructured conversational style and group members would freely offer each other feedback about the latest events of their lives, problems they were encountering, and ideas and feelings they were experiencing. Group members had always told me that they liked this way of working, but as my knowledge of narrative ideas expanded I became less comfortable with some of the taken-for-granted practices of the typical format. For example, while I felt that the use of affirmations and positive feedback like, 'Great job', and 'You were really brave to have pulled that off', were helpful to group members, I didn't see them as contributing to thicker descriptions of the group members' preferred versions of themselves.

I had begun to believe that there was a great potential for group therapy to thicken the group members' descriptions of their lives in ways that would enable them to step into new ways of being. I certainly encouraged group members to talk about how they identified with the person speaking, but initially the ways in which I did this didn't help them to link how they specifically related to the speaker or why they found this identification remarkable. Opportunities to further link the group members' lives in meaningful ways were lost. I wanted to structure the group's time to maximise the authentication of members' identity claims.

I decided to use the reflecting team format in my gay men's therapy group. I was quite familiar with reflecting team methodology, having used it with clients, in the training program in which I teach, and in peer supervision. However, I think what really made me understand the impact that reflecting teams can have was to be on the inside of the work myself. While attending an intensive at Dulwich Centre this past winter, I experienced being the person at the centre of one of the reflecting teams. Through that process I realised how my own experiences of loneliness and suffering while growing up gay were actually expressed in my work as a therapist with other gay men now. I also began to re-appreciate how surviving oppression had given me skills and knowledges that made it possible for me to move beyond just surviving, to a place where I could be patient and loving and strong in all my work as a therapist, and especially in my conversations with other gay men. Seeing how my experience of oppression and self-hatred had been transformed into expressions of love, convinced me that the gay men who consulted me could reconstitute their lives as well. I saw how reflecting team work was one way to create a context in which this could happen.

At first I was concerned that group members might feel disappointed, because fewer members' lives would be at the centre of the evening's conversation. It was after the second or third time that we tried using reflecting teams in the gay men's group that I put my concern to the group and I was reassured. Ed quipped: *I don't want to seem self-centred or anything, but when I'm on the team I'm not just thinking about the other guy. As I listen to you both talk, my mind is full of thoughts about my own life and emotions, and about things that have happened to me. I'm engaged with what he's talking about, but from my own frame of reference, so I don't feel short-changed in anyway at all. In fact, I like doing the group this way better.*

What follows is a description of my most recent practice and my thoughts about it.

**Check-in**

Like most groups, we begin with a brief go-around that allows each member to check-in with the others about how he is doing and any recent developments in his life. It's also a time for group members to signal to the leader if he would like any time to talk that evening. Since it is not always possible for each person's life to be at the centre of the evening's conversation, checking in ensures that everyone at least gets to talk a bit. Group members have told me it is an important part of feeling as if they belong.

Years ago, when I first started this group with my dear friend Fred Wolf, he would always start the next part of the group by saying, 'Who needs air time?' This has become a tradition which gives me a chance to negotiate with the group about who we will be talking with and how to divide the time. Depending on the circumstances, we have found that one or two people can be interviewed in an hour and a half session. It is not at all uncommon for us to focus on just one. Once it is decided whose life will be at the centre, we follow a four-phase interview structure for reflecting teams (White 1995).

I see my role as interviewer and reflecting team facilitator. My job is to create a forum where the expert knowledges of the group members are privileged. My expertise is to build a scaffold for these knowledges to be confirmed. I do not leave it to chance, as I did previously, for the person at the centre's preferred claims about his life to be acknowledged or more thickly described. My role is central, and I do not deny my special knowledge as a facilitator.

**Tellings**

I have come to think that much of the group session involves group members engaging in the 'tellings' of their lives. In order to ensure that the person's life who is now at the centre of the group stays at the centre, and to ensure that the ensuing conversations contribute to lives more thickly described, I offer these following general guidelines to the rest of the group whom I consider to be the witness group or reflecting team. I have found that these guidelines will help to lead the group towards four classes of responses: joining, orientating to mystery, exploring alternative landscapes, and deconstructing one's interests (White 1995).

- Listen very carefully to the story, especially for how it relates to your own experience.
- Notice any images which come up for you from this person's life and from yours.
- Be ready to acknowledge your appreciation for what he is going through.
- Be curious about the developments in this person's life.
- Be tentative in your comments. Use the 'subjunctive mood' and phrases that leave openings for uncertainty: 'I was wondering …' or 'I'm not sure about this but …'
- Be prepared to answer questions about what struck you and why.

These are minimal guidelines to set the stage for a thoughtful and rich team process. With five minutes of training and some occasional coaching, group members have little difficulty doing a fantastic job on the reflecting team. With the team together in one place (in their own small circle off to the side in the same room), I begin a conversation with the person whose life is at the centre. I have what I consider to be a typical narrative-type conversation with him. These types of conversations have been described at length in the literature about narrative therapy. In these conversations I work with the person consulting me to: negotiate an experience-near, particular, non-structuralist definition of the problem or of the alternative story; map the effects of the problem or alternative story on the life of the person; engage in an evaluation of those effects; and encourage the person to justify those evaluations.[1] These types of conversations give people an opportunity to truly engage with the stories of their lives. As active participants, they take a position on their experience and the meaning they make of their lives. In our group I have found that a conversation of a half an hour to forty-five minutes gives the reflecting team group more than enough to reflect on.

What follows is a description of some of the themes that emerge in the tellings that take place in the group. I have also included some typical questions I might ask around these themes. After I have described some of these themes I will explore the ways in which the reflecting processes operate in the group.

### *Externalising homophobia/the influence of heterosexual dominance*

Early in the work it is often useful to externalise homophobia as a way of separating the person from the problem. Frequently people who are gay are surprised to think of themselves as carrying homophobia, but by examining how homophobia has been socially constructed, how they face it in their day-to-day lives (e.g. through silence about the details of their lives, fear of physical harm), they are more clearly able to take a position against homophobia in their lives. It has been useful to think about homophobia as a manifestation of heterosexual dominance as a way of deconstructing how it is a dimension of power woven into the social fabric. Personal descriptions of homophobia, such as 'life in the closet', or 'the shame game', help to make the externalisation more experience-near. By taking a position on the effects of homophobia, a person is able to connect with ways that a self-hating position is not consistent with his own beliefs.

- *How do you see heterosexual dominance influencing your relationships with your co-workers?*
- *Do you find that heterosexual dominance silences you when you are talking with them about what you did with your weekend?*
- *Why is it that homophobia doesn't fit with your dreams for your life?*

***Coming out***

Many of the men who attend the group are 'out', having told their family and friends they are gay. Many of the other group members are extremely scared about letting anyone know about their sexuality. So the very fact that they have even joined the group is discussed as a unique outcome that may be more embracing of an identity as an 'out' person. I have found it necessary to be transparent about my own political belief that being 'out' is better than being in the closet, that being put in the closet is part of the discursive practices of heterosexual dominance. It is important to note that, despite my strong preference for people to be open about their sexuality, the person at the centre needs to decide the pace of his coming out. Being 'out' may make him vulnerable to real physical danger, loss of job or housing and cut-off from family and friends. We also emphasise 'coming out' as a process that never ends and that people in our lives may need time, just as we ourselves did, to adjust to the fact that we are gay.

- *Wow, you came 'out' to your sister! What does that say about the kind of relationship you would like to have with her?*
- *Right in that moment, after you told her about being gay, how did you feel?*
- *How does that fit with how you want to live your life?*

***Oppression breeds depression***

Each June in the annual gay pride parade in our city, a contingent from our group volunteers to march together. Last year one of the group members carried the slogan 'oppression breeds depression' on his picket sign. We have spent many hours in our group talking about the effects of depression in our lives. We have explored how describing the emotional effects of oppression as a clinical symptom obscures the political nature of the so-called disorder. We have examined how being gay in our culture may give rise to 'symptoms' such as feelings of worthlessness and guilt, isolation, depressed mood and even a desire to kill oneself.

- *Have you found that being 'out' to your friends has been a bit of an antidote to the sadness you used to feel when you were around them?*
- *Besides taking Prozac, what else have you been doing to fight against the effects of depression in your life?*

### Monolithic gay culture

This is an expression we made up to describe what has also been referred to as 'internalising the oppressor'. Oftentimes when a gay man comes out, he may expect that, after years of oppression in 'straight culture', he will be welcomed with open arms into the gay world. Instead he may be confronted with a subculture that marginalises certain types of other gays. Older men may feel profoundly disqualified by the huge emphasis on youth and physical fitness that pervades much of gay culture. Transvestites or people who practise sadomasochism may be edited out of portrayed versions of gay life because they do not fit the political ideal that 'we're just like everyone else'.

In the group, the steps toward freedom from oppression are framed as moving away from global or essentialist accounts of people. It is worth noting, however, that gay culture also does offer some ready-made accounts of life for people to step into, such as 'pride', which can be profoundly affirming.

- *How did you claim being forty-six and overweight in the face of such strong stereotypes in the gay community?*
- *How does knowing that the Stonewall riots of 1969 were initiated by drag queens, help you to reclaim your identity as one of them?*

### Relationships

Many of the gay men who consult me speak of having had difficulty developing long-term loving relationships, and I think this is because of the influences of isolation and other negative effects of homophobia. In addition, gay culture has, in general, venerated casual, sexualised relationships. The group is a counterculture that supports preferred descriptions of the person as lovable and as capable of sustaining a long-term loving relationship or any relationship of his choosing. (We do have a rule that group members do not engage in sexual relationships with each other while in the group, not because we're against sex, but because it makes things too complicated in the group.) Group members may find that after 'coming out' they have another 'adolescence', learning about dating and socialising all over again.

- *Regarding relationships, where do you see yourself going in your life now that you've laid this ground work?*
- *How does being more visible as a gay man fit with your dreams for a relationship with another man?*

***Creating/joining community***

Homophobia has cut off gay men from each other. An alternative story of connection has these men stepping into membership with each other in political action groups, AIDS service organisations and social networks. Whether it's working with others to pass equal protection laws or going to a ballroom dancing group, joining lives around shared themes expands the witnesses to preferred claims that the men have about their identities and lives.

- *Now that you're leaving the group, how do you think your friends at the gay newspaper will continue to support you?*
- *Where else do you find what you've found here?*

## Retellings of the tellings

After the group member at the centre of the conversation has completed his telling, this is when the rest of the group reflects. At the Family Institute of Maine we have experimented with many different spatial arrangements for reflecting teams and have decided that in general, when circumstances allow it, having the team in a separate space and connected by a one-way mirror or closed circuit television has the best outcomes. This clearly delineates the performers from the audience and heightens the ceremonial aspects of the work. However, for the work described in this paper, I have only been able to use one room. We form two distinct clusters in the same room, and I move between the two over the course of the process.

We follow the format that most narrative reflecting teams do – each person speaking from his own experience about the conversation they have just witnessed. In the gay men's group I have found that the linking of lives around shared themes happens quite readily with little intervention on my part. I have a fairly light touch as a facilitator at this point. Again I see my role as providing a scaffold. My primary role during the retellings is to act as an interviewer to ensure that the reflections are linked back to the life of the person at the centre, to deconstruct comments with the aim of further linking lives, and to unpack unquestioned assumptions. (This is especially helpful if a group member has lapsed into giving advice.) Here are a few examples of the types of questions I might ask:

- *Ed, you said that you were impressed that John got up and delivered the eulogy at this father's funeral. What in your own history made that seem like such a huge accomplishment to you?*
- *What other things did you hear John say that led you to see that as an impressive event? Do you have any guesses about what made it possible for him to take that step?*
- *When Bill talked about telling his boss at work that he was gay, did you have a sense about some of the things he was overcoming in making that revelation?*
- *Given your own experience in 'coming out' as gay, what do you imagine he was struggling against in that moment?*
- *Alan, why do you think that, of all the people in this group who heard Dan telling us about going for an HIV antibody test, you found it remarkable? Why did it strike a chord for you?*
- *You seem quite certain that monogamous relationships are the best way for people to go. Am I right about that? What in your experience has made you so convinced of that as a value?*

- *Larry, you were talking about a soaring eagle just a moment ago. Can you say what is was about what John was telling us about that brought this image to you?*

The focus of the team's reflections and my questions create a process where people's lives are more richly described. The men in this group have often experienced themselves as invisible because their lives are dominated by isolation, and often have a sense of their identities as spoiled. For them, these reflecting teams are an opportunity to re-engage with themselves as deeply connected with others and to be embraced by an account of themselves as people deserving to be cherished and understood. As a result of the team acting as a witness in this way, the life of the person at the centre becomes multi-voiced, connected to many others around their preferred claims about their identities or histories. The difficult tasks of resisting oppression and becoming visible are supported.

In this way the conversations within the group become a process of community building. As Sharon Welch describes, *the ability to resist – the continual reminders that it is possible and worthwhile – is sustained by the creation of alternative structures, by a community in which love that compels and sustains resistance is fully expressed* (1990, p.80). My hope is that the group serves this sort of role in the lives of its members.

## A note regarding applause

I would like to add here that when a team member does make a reflection that might fall under the category of 'applause'(White 1997, p.97), it is easy enough to remedy. I think these types of comments can be expected in the thinning discourse of popular culture. I make it my job to help to deconstruct these reflections when they come up, ensuring that I do so in ways that do not shame or discourage. If someone says, 'That was absolutely fabulous what he did', I will follow up by asking something like, 'From what John told us about his own hopes for his life, what gives you the idea that he would evaluate that development as fabulous?' or 'Say, Richard, of all the people who responded to that part of what John was saying, why was it you that noticed it and remarked upon it?' These sorts of questions invite Richard to talk about the developments in John's life in terms of his own life, and encourage a discussion around joint purposes, hopes and dreams.

It has taken me a few years (at least) to expand beyond mere affirmations and to restrain myself from sharing my own evaluations with those who consult me. In these teams I have come to expect applause, so I just work with it when it comes.

## Retellings of the retellings

What has stood out to me in my work with the gay men's group is the way that the telling is made more real by the retellings, how the retellings expand on the boundaries of the tellings. After the reflecting team has offered their reflections, I return to sit with the person who is consulting the team and interview him about his experience of the reflecting team. I have found a good way to get started is to orient the interview to three questions:

1. Among the things you heard from the team, what stood out to you as helpful or important?
2. Was there anything that just didn't fit for you?
3. Is there anything you would like to do differently or follow up on as a result of this conversation?

Of course, there are at least a million other possible questions. I have found that these types of questions generally work to continue to link the life of the person at the centre of the conversation with those on the reflecting team. At this point in the process the person generally experiences himself as profoundly embraced by the preferred descriptions of his life.

This part of the consultation is also a time to ask other follow-up questions aimed at further linking the group members around shared purposes and dreams:

- *How did Alan's reflections speak to you about your hopes for the future with your new partner? What was it that he said that rang true for you?*
- *Why do you think what Jim was saying about how he handled a similar situation with his wife fit so well for you?*

## Wrapping up

The last part of the evening is a less structured conversation which gives people a chance to talk all together about the process and to debrief a bit. Often a team member will talk about what another member's reflections meant to him or they will offer words of encouragement or thanks to the person who has been at the centre. It is also an opportunity for them to interview me about my experience of the process. They may ask me why I asked a certain question or took a certain direction in the interview. I may take the opportunity to speak about how the work shapes my own life, the contributions of the group to my sense of myself as a therapist, as a person and as another gay man. We always give the person at the centre a chance to have the last say – really to say anything he wishes, and then we all say goodbye. Many of the fellows in the group go out for coffee afterward and get together during the intervening week to take walks together, go to the movies, and so forth.

## Saying goodbye

When someone leaves the group, we make an event of it. Our ceremony for saying goodbye is for each of the group members to acknowledge how the person who is leaving has contributed to his life and what his connection to him has meant. The person leaving also speaks with the other members about these kinds of contributions.

Paul was leaving the group after eight months. He had recently come 'out' to his wife, got divorced, and then had come 'out' to all of his colleagues in graduate school. He also reported that he had stepped into an identity as a gay man that he felt at one with and that corresponded with his desire to accept himself, enjoy his sexuality, and to be loved by those around him.

> *You guys have all been part of a time in my life that was really hard, even more difficult than having cancer when I was nineteen – at least I had support around that. For thirty-five years I had felt really alone in my sexuality and now something has shifted. For all that time I really hated myself. I felt disgusting for having sexual thoughts about other men. I was*

> *feeding into all of society's stuff about being gay ... In the past six months there's been a huge shift. I love myself now. I accept who I am and how I am – everything about me. I accept the fact that I have hazel eyes and I'm balding and I'm gay. It's all part of me. What made that transition easier is that you guys accepted it first before I did. You made me realise I'm not the piece of crap I thought I was.*
>
> *I remember when I was still struggling and I typed in a message into my computer – 'I'm a 35 year old man looking for a support group'. It was hard to type in that message. Chris, you responded and you gave me your information. Boy, was I really scared just typing that in and hitting send. It was acknowledging something about myself. Returning your call to me, that was also acknowledging something. Coming to see you was acknowledging some more, and it was really overwhelming. I was really depressed at the time, but it was a real turning point. I am glad you were all there to get my message.*

Regarding the use of reflecting teams in the group, Paul said:

> *For me, I really liked that process. It just made things more real. I liked the intensity of it. In a traditional setting, where everyone says what they have to say, there is something too quick. Without the team too many things can be missed. One person would say something, then someone would say something right after, and someone after that. You don't get as much that way. With the reflecting team, where we sit and actually reflect, you can plug into whatever the person has been talking about and pull up in your mind whatever's been happening in your life that's similar. The process drives itself. It's a different energy.*

**Acknowledgements**

This paper is dedicated to my dear friend Fred Wolf who started and co-led this group with me for five years. He died two days after Christmas last year at the age of 76. I listened to Sarah McLachlan on my laptop pretty much continuously as I wrote this paper, remembering him. She sings 'I will remember you. Will you remember me? Don't let your life pass you by. Weep not for the memories.'

In November and December 1998 I attended the Level I and II Intensives with Michael White at Dulwich Centre in Adelaide, South Australia, where, among many other wonderful happenings, my work in this group with gay men was richly acknowledged.

Finally, I want to acknowledge the contributions to this work by the men in my group. I am amazed by how patient they have been with me as I continue to learn. I have used some of their first names in quotations throughout this paper. I am grateful to them all.

**Note**

1. This orientation to therapeutic conversations has been greatly influenced by Michael White's Statement of Position Micro-map (Dulwich Centre intensive training course, 1998).

# 18

# Weaving new stories over the phone

## A narrative approach to a Gay Switchboard

by

Bill Logan

*In the Wellington Gay Welfare Group/Gay Switchboard, we have developed our own very powerful traditions of how to support men in the process of coming out. These are community-based traditions that are heavily influenced by methods of gaylines around the world, and owe a great deal to our origins in the post-Stonewall gay liberation movement of the late 1970s. This paper describes a framework for the work that we do.*

**Coming out**

Coming out is a process in which a person 'rewrites' the story they have about themself. Before the process starts, they have a self-story which is more or less heterosexual, a story which they have absorbed from the world around them. It is a story which has them living as a heterosexual, known to their family and friends and workmates as heterosexual, and which predicts a heterosexual future. But for those people who call the Switchboard, this heterosexual story doesn't fit – perhaps they never quite felt that it fitted, or perhaps rather suddenly it has started to feel very uncomfortable. Often the contradiction between their sexual and emotional desires and the heterosexual story has led to great anguish and confusion, perhaps even for a prolonged period. Coming out is a process of writing compulsory heterosexuality out of the story, and other forms of sexual and emotional expression into it.

As workers on the Switchboard, our role in the process by which callers rewrite the stories of their lives and sexual identities is pretty modest. The callers do the work, usually turning to us only as a preliminary audience, for reassurance, or perhaps when they get stuck. Even though our role is modest, the more we understand, the more we are able to assist the process. In this paper, I'll describe some of the questions we ask to try to assist our callers remake their stories. I don't in any way want to imply that there is a series of stages or steps in our counselling work, for this is not the case. For a start, most callers will do much re-storying without our help and will turn to us only at particular points. Even if we were present for the whole coming out re-storying process, it is never tidy or linear. Coming out is more like a process of weaving back and forth between the old story and the new story, between the past, the present and the future, between feelings and ideas.

While it is in the intense phase of coming out that the Switchboard is most often helpful, coming out is not a process that comes to an end – it continues throughout life. We go on developing, making ourselves, refining our stories. Although this paper is geared to Switchboard callers who are in their intense primary 'coming out' phase, I believe its underlying ideas can be applied far more widely. Furthermore, there are some similarities to narrative therapy which are explored below and in the table at the end of this paper.

## 1. Queer listening

More than anything else in our work, we have always stressed the importance of active, empathetic *listening*. It is our prime job to be a good audience both for the old 'problem-saturated' story, and for the early editions of an exciting new story. Our listening, then, enhanced by a real care for our callers and a sense of empathy which comes from having had some parallel experiences ourselves, is an extremely significant element of what we bring to our conversations on the Switchboard.

The kind of listening which has informed our training sessions is known in the counselling literature as 'Rogerian' (named after the influential psychologist Carl Rogers) or as client-centred listening. My understanding of Rogerian or client-centred listening, and what it has offered to me as a worker, is an acknowledgment of the significance of *reflecting* back a caller's feelings to them, staying where they are at in a conversation and playing a role of clarifying and summarising where the caller is coming from. These have all been extremely powerful tools and significant philosophical orientations to the conversations we share with callers.

In practice, our listening does something more than reflection. Our callers contact us because we are a gay agency. It is likely that we have been selected as the audience for these stories *because* we are gay. Typically a caller early in the process of coming out has a life predominantly defined by heterosexuality, but has some fantasy or activity which contradicts that definition. As there are few places within the mainstream culture where respectful audiences can be found to non-heterosexual stories, and as the caller has chosen to ring a Gay Switchboard, we feel we have special job to listen for the non-heterosexual and emotional desires, the exceptions to the dominant heterosexual story, and to provide a chance for the meaning of these experiences to be explored. This is what the narrative approach calls *deconstructive listening to the problem-saturated story*, and which we could call *queer listening*. Queer listening is characterised by a special kind of curiosity. We are especially interested in those elements of the story that do not fit within a compulsory heterosexuality. We listen to the heartache, we empathise with the sense of confusion our callers may be experiencing, we reflect back the grief they feel, but we also maintain a curiosity which seeks to make possible an expanded exploration of the gay element of the story.

## 2. Externalising homophobia[1]

Perhaps the most valuable practical tool that narrative therapy has offered us is that of *externalisation*, but even this technique is not entirely new to our work. The basic theoretical idea of the Switchboard has always been that the problems our callers have are not to be understood as something to do with their sexual feelings but instead are due to homophobia – the fear of homosexuality which still pervades society. It is often useful to explain this concept of homophobia quite directly to callers, and it is commonly quite dramatically liberatory for them to hear 'their' problems talked about as being an outside force with its own name – a thing to be dealt with rather than something wrong within the caller himself. Once we have introduced the idea of homophobia, we can often relate the experiences that a caller talks about to that idea. Usually after a while they start doing this for themselves.

*Caller*: I was always afraid I might be called gay when I was a teenager.

*Switchboarder*: Where do you think this fear came from?

*Caller*: Well – my family would have been pretty down on gays. And there was a lot of anti-gay stuff at school.

*Switchboarder*: Anti-gay stuff? What would you call this? We often call it homophobia[2]. Does that fit for you?

*Caller*: It was a homophobic place.

*Switchboarder*: It's a bit like a disease, isn't it? The fear of gayness. Would you say that there was a lot of this anti-gay stuff, this homophobia at school?

*Caller*: Yes, it was pretty bad.

*Switchboarder*: Can you tell me a bit about that?

*Caller*: Well there was graffiti in the toilets. And I had the reputation of being a poofter. I don't know why. I was always getting hassled. I hated school.

*Switchboarder*: So this homophobia was pretty hurtful, then? What did you do about it?

*Caller*: I just kept to myself.

*Switchboarder*: Would you say the homophobia was very isolating for you, then?

*Caller*: Yeah.

Switchboarder: Tell me something about how you first became aware that you weren't completely heterosexual?

*Caller*: Well I suppose in the third and forth form I felt sexually attracted to boys, and I was scared of that – I never did anything about it.

*Switchboarder*: Would you say it was the homophobia that made you afraid of being gay?

*Caller*: Yes I suppose so.

Narrative therapy trains counsellors in a general habit of inviting externalising conversations about problems. If someone complains of being ashamed, the counsellor will separate the shame from the identity of the client by a manner of talking about the shame as an entity outside the person, asking where the shame came from, what makes it bigger or smaller, and so on. If someone complains of feeling guilty, the counsellor might ask what conditions make the guilt worse, or even start to talk of the guilt as if it were a person, asking if the guilt has any allies, for example. So, narrative therapists will seek to name a problem as if it were an outside agent affecting a person's life, thereby helping the client escape from the sense of being totally consumed and controlled by the problem, and making it seem more possible for them to have some sense of choices in how he or she deals with the problem.

In some ways we have been using this technique of externalising homophobia right from the time the Switchboard started. We have done similarly with other concepts such as 'heterosexism', 'macho values', 'the closet', and so on. We could, however, probably be a lot more persistent than we usually are with questions which help people see that homophobia comes from outside themselves.

Some possible lines of questions include:

- *In what ways does homophobia control your life?*

- *How does homophobia hurt you? What other effects does it have?*
- *What does homophobia steal from you? What pleasures does it take away from you?*
- *What does homophobia tell you about yourself? Has homophobia robbed you of pride in yourself?*
- *If you look back a year, do you think that homophobia was a stronger influence then than it is now, or weaker?*

### 3. Relative influence questioning

The externalisation of the problem is made more significant in narrative therapy by a process called *relative influence questioning* which involves two kinds of questions, one kind which maps the influence of the problem on the person, and another kind which involves mapping the influence of people on the problem.

We are applying this technique when on the one hand we draw out the effects that homophobia has on a caller, or on the other hand we draw out ways the caller has been able to hide or escape from the influences of homophobia, or resist it and fight back against it.

*Caller*: I know that I want to go to the sauna, but I don't know if I have the courage.

*Switchboarder*: What stops you going, do you think?

*Caller*: I dunno. I guess I'm afraid of what it will mean if I go there.

*Switchboarder*: I'm really interested in this fear, and how it stops you doing what you know you want to do. What would you call it? What would you call this fear?

*Caller*: I dunno.

*Switchboarder*: We could call it the Fear? Or a fear of gayness? Or homophobia? Or something else? What do you think?

*Caller*: I'm worried about what I'll think, I'm worried about how others will react. I guess that's homophobia.

*Switchboarder*: And so, this homophobia, has it stopped you doing other things that you know you want to do? Does homophobia stop you from having any sex with men at all?

*Caller*: Well I told you about the times when I was drunk with my mate.

*Switchboarder*: What about when you're sober? Have you ever had any sex with guys when you're sober? What about in your imagination? Do you ever *think* about sex with guys when you are sober?

*Caller*: Well yeah, I think about sex with guys quite often, but it makes me feel very guilty.

*Switchboarder*: Is this the homophobia again? Does it make you feel bad about your fantasies?

*Caller*: Yeah.

*Switchboarder*: But it isn't so strong that you stop the fantasies?

*Caller*: No. Not usually.

*Switchboarder*: How do you think you managed to keep the homophobia at bay long enough to continue having these dreams, these fantasies?

*Caller*: I don't know. I guess I just enjoy them. They kind of have a life of their own …

Some lines of relative influence questioning include:

***The effect of the homophobia on the caller***

- *What kinds of things does homophobia convince you that you should do? What kinds of things does it stop you doing?*
- *How does the homophobia prevent you from going to the sauna / gay bar / coming out group?*

***The effect of the caller on homophobia***

- *When you were growing up, did you have any ways of hiding from homophobia in your family or at school?*
- *Were there any particular times that you can remember when you managed to lessen homophobia's influence?*
- *What have you noticed what helps make you stronger in dealing with homophobia?*
- *Who are the people in your life who might be allies against homophobia?*

## 4. Social critique

Inherent in the Switchboard approach is a criticism of a society in which the heterosexual norm is so strongly entrenched. The socially dominant stories of mythical heterosexual bliss are at times the source of our callers' ill-fitting personal stories, and so it is these social stories, as much as the callers' personal problem-saturated stories, which must be unravelled.

Whether it is called social critique or deconstruction of the dominant discourse, what we are doing is helping our callers stand outside the general presumption that heterosexuality is the norm by which all other forms of sexual expression are to be judged. It is not usually useful to offer callers long theoretical explanations about sex-role stereotyping in the patriarchal bourgeois nuclear family! Finding ways to remain sensitive to where our callers are at is important. As a service, however, we do have clear ideas about the sociology of the family, about the role of dominant constructions of masculinity, about the traditional subordination of women, and so on. Our ethical beliefs about these issues inform the questions we ask, such as:

- *Looking back, you've spoken about how homophobia was present in your childhood. Do you think homophobia is present in many people's childhood?*
- *What does homophobia think men should be like in this society?*

- *How does homophobia influence how some people act? What does it have them doing?*
- *What do you think are the effects of homophobia? For men's lives, women's lives, children's lives?*
- *What kinds of things might be done to make homophobia in society weaker?*
- *What do you imagine a world would be like without homophobia?*

## 5. Exploring sparkling moments

No matter how problem-saturated the story is, there are always exceptional events – moments and actions which are inconsistent with the problem-saturated story, developments in which the problem has not been in control. Narrative workers call these exceptional events *unique outcomes* or *sparkling moments*, and it is from these that new preferred stories are created.

On the Switchboard we explore those moments of fantasy and activity which defy the heterosexual story. We invite callers to talk about remembered childhood thoughts of being 'different', about boyhood camaraderie, about pubescent consciousness of homosexual desire, about early same-sex sexual experiences and fantasies, and about times they as young men stood outside the dominant constructions of heterosexual masculinity.

Some starting questions might include:

- *Tell me about times when you have not allowed homophobia to control you.*
- *What were your first victories against homophobia? How did they happen?*
- *Have you ever fantasised about having sex with men? How did you push the homophobia back enough to let you have those fantasies?*
- *Have you ever had sex with a man? How did you manage to escape the control of homophobia sufficiently for that?*

One of the very best things we can do for our callers is to invite them to catalogue these sparkling moments. But we are not satisfied with sketchy catalogue-style descriptions – we are interested in details. We want to find ways in which little moments can be expanded into sub-plots and linked to other sub-plots. A story lives in the details, and we seek in conversations to build a richness of description of such moments and a relating of such moments to other aspects of life.

So we are interested in where and when and with whom. We are interested in the colour of the other guy's hair and what he was wearing and the music that was playing. We are interested in the kind of personality he had and what his lifestyle was. We are interested in how the caller reacted to the event and the impact it had on the caller's sleep and his work and everything else in his life. We are particularly interested in the details of the meaning of the event for the caller – what the event(s) spoke to him about his life and hopes and dreams[3].

We are interested in discovering a variety of *kinds* of sparkling moment or exceptional event. These are not just sexual events. Often the key influence of homophobia is to prevent the caller from disclosing his homosexuality to anyone else. It is often this that is most bothering the caller. There are always exceptions to this aspect of the problem, too – there are sparkling moments of disclosure in even the most closeted of stories. This is not so strange to us – we frequently find ourselves asking a first-time caller to consider what significance the act of calling the Switchboard has had for them. Very often the first call is a courageous exception to the old story in which homophobia has turned important parts of life into 'dirty secrets'. The first call is often a sparkling moment to explore and build upon.

The first call can often also be used retrospectively as in the following example:

*Switchboarder*: Can you think back to the first time you rang us? Were you thinking about making that first call for very long before you did?

*Caller*: Yes, for a few weeks.

*Switchboarder*: Was it hard to build up the courage to ring?

*Caller*: Yes, I was pretty shit-scared.

*Switchboarder*: Thinking back, can you explain what that fear was all about, then?

*Caller*: I guess I was afraid that by calling you I was kind of giving in to being gay. I was afraid of being gay.

*Switchboarder*: So calling us was in some way standing up to that fear? How did you manage to get it together to call us? How did you overcome the fear about gayness?

*Caller*: Well I figured that I better do something. I figured I couldn't live the rest of my life paralysed by fear.

*Switchboarder*: So you knew you didn't want to live a life in fear. Is that right? Can you explain to me a bit more how that meant you were able to ring?

*Caller*: Well I had been thinking about sex with men for years, and I'd never done anything about it. I felt really stuck. I sort of had to ring you guys, or I thought I'd never do anything for my whole life.

*Switchboarder*: So ringing was not only standing up to fear about being gay, but also standing up to a fear of not doing anything with your life? Is that right?

*Caller*: Yes, I thought I had to start having a life sometime.

*Switchboarder*: So making the call was like taking a step towards having a life? Is that right?

*Caller*: Yeah.

Having got to this point in the conversation, the Switchboarder could then explore what taking a 'step towards having a life' meant for the caller, whether it was good thing, if so why, and what he thought it said about him that he could take that step. This conversation would lead into considerations of what the caller wanted for this life, his hopes and how calling the Switchboard was reaching out to those dreams. Whenever a sparkling moment is identified, it can be used as an opportunity to ask questions that invite the caller into considering how these moments influence his sense of his own identity. We are interested in exploring in detail the meanings of sparkling moments in callers' lives.

## 6. Trying on labels

As a new story starts to develop which is not dominated by homophobia – a story in which there is some room for non-heterosexuality – it can be helpful to start to 'fix' the new story with a name. It is not up to us what label of sexuality our callers decide to wear, and we are relaxed about the likelihood that their label-preference will change. It's also fine if callers prefer not to wear any label at all. But inviting questions which pose choices about self-descriptions can help people make decisions in story-lines, and can help them construct a self-description that fits for them.

- *From what you've told me about your life and what you want for your life, does the word heterosexual fully fit for you?*
- *Do you have words that for now might describe you better?*
- *What would it mean in your life if you started using the word* [insert caller's word] *to yourself right now?*

## 7. Detailing the action

Telling and retelling the story of coming to terms with their sexuality helps the caller expand it and make it richer, and that expansion and enrichment can be enhanced by focusing on the story in different ways. Narrative therapists make a distinction between what they call the *landscape of action* and the *landscape of consciousness*[4]. The landscape of action concerns what is *done*, or (which may for many purposes be as important) what is imagined, whereas the landscape of consciousness is concerned with the meanings of these events or imaginings. In the context of coming out, the landscape of action refers to homosexual fantasy and experience, disclosure of homosexuality to other people, and such life-changes as leaving a marriage.

- *Tell me something about how gay feelings have been part of your life in the past. When did you first notice gayness? What was it like to notice that?*
- *What things have you done towards having the sexual life you want?*
- *What was the first step you took?*
- *Who was the first person you told?*

The action-line of a story goes from the past, through the present, to the future. Obviously a great deal of attention will be given to current activities and a large part of the counselling process might well be about what happened just last night, how to overcome today's obstacle, or the fears about disclosing one's homosexuality to a best friend tomorrow. Very often a lot of Switchboard discussion is about the *now*. We are also aware of the importance of accumulating detail around histories that will assist callers deal with their present circumstances. For example, we often try to explore *past* events which speak to a willingness on the part of the caller to resist compulsory heterosexuality and homophobia. These past examples of actions often enable a stronger sense of identity in the present. What we could perhaps give more attention to in our work is development of the future of callers' stories:

- *If you managed to resist homophobia effectively, how do you think your life would be?*
- *In a year's time, do you think your life will be the same as it is now, or do you think that you will have taken steps to push homophobia out of your life?*

## 8. Developing the landscape of consciousness

A story is not just a series of events, one after the other. The point about a story is that it tells events according to patterns and meanings, and so the development of a new story requires a development in what narrative therapists describe as the *landscape of consciousness*. It is in this domain that people have knowledge about themselves, in which they have their values and beliefs, and in which they see their own stories connected to wider cultural discourses.

On the Switchboard we are sensitive to a development in our callers of self-esteem, a sense of the inherent goodness of gayness, a feeling of pride. One of the ways we do this is to ask questions that invite callers to reflect on the meaning of certain acts or steps that they have taken.

For example, when callers retell events from their past in which they resisted the effects of homophobia and/or compulsory heterosexuality, we are able to ask about the meanings of these events.

- *What do you believe it says about you that you were able to take this step?*
- *Who else would recognise in you the attributes that this step required?*

It is also significant that many callers find a better equilibrium in their lives as gay people to the extent that they have thought about and decided where they stand in relation to the larger issues of gay community life, sexual politics, gay liberation and queer theory.

At various points in our connection with a caller, conversations around the following kinds of themes might be appropriate:

- *Has your sense of yourself as a person changed as your acceptance of your sexuality has increased?*
- *What does it tell you about yourself that you are increasingly having the strength to resist homophobia in your life?*
- *As you live a life which is more and more free of homophobia, how do you think you will see yourself as a person? Is your pride in yourself decreasing or increasing ?*
- *How do you understand this growing pride in yourself? Is it in anyway connected to your ideas about gay liberation? Queer consciousness?*

## 9. Using gay cultural resources

While every person's story is unique, the uniqueness is largely in the combination of the elements. Many of the elements of all of our stories are borrowed from a huge variety of sources. We use bits and pieces from our cultural environment, transforming them along the way. The way we understand ourselves and events, the way we tell them, and the way we perform our stories is derived from the cultural resources around us. In transcending a problem-saturated story, the richer our cultural experience in relevant areas, the better the possibilities for new stories which transcend the problems. Of course there arc some areas in which the resources available in the wider discourses of the culture are more developed than others. Narrative therapists have taken to building cultural resources for their clients in some areas, such as bulimia and anorexia. There are various examples of therapists building archives – collecting accounts of clients' struggles against their problems and accounts of their successes – so that clients through their documents can help each other and be helped by each other[5].

On the Switchboard we don't have to build an archive – there already exists a rich body of gay cultural resources, and Switchboard has always recommended gay novels, coming out memoirs, history and film to callers. It's not all high-culture, either. We are not ashamed to talk about gay icons in the world of entertainment or rumours about sporting greats. Videos that celebrate gay sex are often also significant resources. It is in reaction to all these sorts of materials that callers develop their own story-lines.

We try to take care, however, to guard against any sense that the cultural resources we recommend are prescriptive of ways of being. We don't believe that any resource should tell a caller how he should live his life or pattern his sexual interactions. It is often as useful for a caller to be able to say to himself 'This is NOT me' as it is to be able to say 'This IS me'. We try to convey this belief in all of our conversations.

## 10. Using peer-groups

An important part of coming out is the development of a network of gay friends, whose roles importantly include story-exchange. To some extent this can be organised or even ritualised. Consciousness-raising groups were a feature of the post-Stonewall gay liberation period. These unstructured, non-hierarchical groups of men, all of whom were in various stages of coming out, provided a forum for the sharing of thoughts and experiences. They were a place where stories of growing up could be shared, a sense of injustice expressed, and where comradeship and support could be given to one another. This tradition continues in the coming out groups and newcomers groups which we have facilitated over the years, and in the Icebreakers Organisation for young gay men which we are currently involved with.

Narrative therapists use a number of different methods to involve peers in the process of re-making identities. Building upon the work of other family therapists, they talk about the usefulness of *reflecting teams* – which listen to a discussion between the client and a counsellor and then reflect on what that discussion brings up for them. It is found that the client can enrich her or his story from these kind of reflections[6]. Narrative therapists have also developed *leagues of problem-fighters*[7], such as anti-bulimia leagues, which link people with common problems and common experiences together. In these leagues each person can be the adviser of others, as well as a learner from others, connections can be made and a sense of community achieved.

Coming out groups fulfil many of the purposes of both reflecting teams and leagues of problem-fighters. Participants tell their stories, their stories impact on an audience of peers, and that impact in turn impacts back on the teller, and the story is refined. The next telling will be just a little bit different, perhaps parts will be told with a little more self-confidence, perhaps parts will be told with a slightly different meaning or significance. Participants hear the stories of others, and parts of those stories seem relevant to themselves. Stories become linked, and as they do the sense of isolation begins to diminish.

## 11. Coming out into the world

It is one thing to tell the new story to a Switchboarder or in a peer group, but telling it in the wider world has a different significance. Narrative therapists place great store in recruiting an audience for the new story and spreading it – *spreading the news,* as they say.[8]

This is significant for many reasons. In the first place, the audience, as a result of hearing the new story, changes its expectations of the teller, which makes it easier for the teller to live and perform the new story. This is something we are familiar with. If you tell Mum and Dad or your workmates that you're gay, even if they react negatively, you're no longer going to need to pretend you have a girlfriend and you're going to find it easier to get on with having a gay life.

In the second place, narrative therapists value spreading the new story because the teller gets feedback from the audience, and this feedback leads to further extensions of the story. The reactions of family and friends to coming out stories become integral parts of the coherence of coming out stories in their later retellings.

In this way coming out involves *performing* a new story in the wider world. These performances occur in many different theatres of life – from one's friendship and family networks, to membership of gay organisations, to gay commercial venues, to the privacy of one's bedroom.

We try to provide conversational support as callers begin to perform their newly crafted identities.

- *Have there been times when you have displayed your gayness?*
- *What were these times like? What does it mean to you that you chose to do this?*
- *Are you interested in telling other people about these stories of your life?*
- *Who would you like to tell apart from me?*
- *What part could we play in supporting this process?*

**Reflections**

Working in the Switchboard has been a significant part of my life now for 18 years. It is difficult to articulate quite what it has meant and continues to mean. It brings a sense of gratification for playing some useful part in the lives of callers but there is much more than this. The concerns of callers inform my own continuing journey but there is much more than this also. There is something sustaining for me in being a part of a group of gay men working together on a valuable project. Like any organisation, we have had our ups and downs, and our disputes – petty and profound. But the Switchboard is a pool of men whom I believe to be remarkable. Jerome (my former partner who died some years ago) was a leading member. Rangimoana (my new partner) has recently joined. Many of my best friends are involved or have been. And when there has been something important to do in this town – to run a campaign for homosexual law reform or start the fight against AIDS – it has been from among Switchboarders that so much of the energy has come. How else to describe what these people mean to me? They have been a significant part of my life now for 18 years.

## Acknowledgements

This paper was first written in mid-1999 for the Wellington Gay Welfare Group and its Gay Switchboard, which I have worked with since 1982. Formal training in the Gay Switchboard had mostly centred on a client-centred Rogerian approach, and this paper was intended to show how in fact our approach was informed also by gay liberation ideas current in the post-Stonewall years which had led us unknowingly to adopt some of the content of narrative therapy. A second intention was to show how our practice could be enriched by a fuller and more conscious engagement with that approach.

A version of the paper was subsequently published as 'Weaving new stories over the phone: a narrative approach to a gay switchboard', *Gecko, a journal of deconstruction and narrative ideas in therapeutic practice*, 1999, Vol.3. That publication included valuable reflection of the paper by Zoy Kazan, Christopher Behan, Claire Ralfs and Patrick O'Leary. I wish to thank all these people for their contributions. I also want to thank Gene Combs, Dominic Davies, Ian MacEwan, Antony McFelin, David Semp, and Bob Trett, and particularly David Denborough (staff writer at Dulwich Centre Publications), who made useful suggestions, and all the members of the Gay Switchboard over the years.


### Notes

1. To read more about externalising conversations and the other narrative ideas described in this paper see Epston, D. & White, M. (1992): *Experience, Contradiction, Narrative & Imagination.* Adelaide: Dulwich Centre Publications.
2. I am aware that in this call the Switchboarder makes a deliberate decision to invite an externalisation of homophobia. Other concepts could have been used, for instance 'anti-gay prejudice' or the words of the caller 'anti-gay stuff'. The decision to externalise homophobia is a political and deliberate one. Homophobia was the key historic externalisation of emergent gay culture after Stonewall that enabled and continues to enable gay people to separate themselves from the effects of dominant attitudes to same-sex sexuality.
3. In asking questions about particularities, we take care that we are seeking details of the meaning of the events for the caller, not just for details of events. This is especially important when talking about sexuality, for any probing for information about another person's sexual activities can be experienced very negatively. We take care to ensure that the conversations are going in helpful directions by asking the caller if these are good things to talk about, and by constantly enquiring about the

meaning of events for the caller so that the conversation is centering the experience of the caller at all times.

4. See White, M. 1991: 'Deconstruction and therapy.' *Dulwich Centre Newsletter,* 3. Reprinted in Epston, D. & White, M. (1992): *Experience, Contradiction, Narrative & Imagination.* Adelaide: Dulwich Centre Publications.
5. See Epston, D. & White, M. 1990: 'Consulting your consultants: The documentation of alternate knowledges.' *Dulwich Centre Newsletter*, No.4. Reprinted in Epston, D. & White, M. (1992): *Experience, Contradiction, Narrative & Imagination.* Adelaide: Dulwich Centre Publications.
6. See Gecko 1999, Vol.2. Special Issue on 'Reflecting teams'.
7. See Grieves, L. 1999: 'From beginning to start: The Vancouver Anti-Anorexia Anti-Bulimia League.' *Gecko*, Vol.2.
8. See Gecko 1999, Vol.2. Special Issue on 'Reflecting teams'.

| Switchboard tradition | Narrative therapy |
|---|---|
| **1. Queer listening** | |
| • Listening, reflection and summarising<br>• Empathy (enhanced by elements of shared story between helper & helped)<br>• Congruence or honesty<br>• Caring or unconditional positive regard<br>• Special attention to elements which contradict the heterosexual story | Deconstructive listening for gaps and contradictions while exploring the problem-saturated story.<br><br>Being the audience for the first tellings of the new preferred story. |
| **2. Externalising homophobia** | |
| Talking about<br>• homophobia<br>• heterosexism<br>• closet<br>• macho values<br>• social expectations | Externalising problems as if they are outside agents affecting a person's life, rather than part of the identity of the person. |
| **3. Relative influence questioning** | |
| • Discussing the effects of homophobia on caller<br>• Discussing the ways the caller has had<br>    • of hiding from homophobia<br>    • of resisting homophobia | • Mapping the influence of the problem on the person<br>• Mapping the influence of the person on the problem |

| Switchboard tradition | Narrative therapy |
|---|---|
| **4. Social critique** | |
| Developing a critique of hetero-normative society (homophobia, sex-role stereotyping, etc.) | Deconstructing the dominant discourse. |
| **5. Exploring sparkling moments** | |
| Affirming the caller's courage in phoning Switchboard<br>Exploring past homosexual experiences and thoughts | Exploring events which are outside the control of the problem (sparkling moments/unique outcomes). |
| **6. Trying on the labels** | |
| Trying on new labels (homosexual,<br>gay, queer, bisexual) | Establishing a name for the new and preferred story. |
| **7. Detailing the action** | |
| Telling and retelling coming out stories with attention to fantasy, activity, disclosure and lifestyle:<br>• past<br>• present<br>• future | Telling and retelling the preferred story with attention to its development in the landscape of action. |
| **8. Developing the landscape of consciousness** | |
| Discussing coming out stories with attention to self-knowledge, values, beliefs, worldview, theory, and philosophy. | Discussing the preferred story with attention to its development in the landscape of consciousness. |

| **Switchboard tradition** | **Narrative therapy** |
|---|---|
| **9. Using gay cultural resources** | |
| Use of gay novels, film, pornography, history, heroic figures, etc. | Use of resources from other clients and archives. |
| **10. Using peer groups** | |
| • Icebreakers<br>• Newcomers groups<br>• Gay Dads<br>• Acquiring gay friends | • Reflecting teams<br>• Leagues of problem-fighters |
| **11. Coming out into the world** | |
| • Disclosing gayness to friends and family<br>• Developing an openly gay lifestyle | • Recruiting an audience and spreading the news<br>• Performing the preferred story |

# 19

# A reflection

from

*Zoy Kazan*

It is clear to me on reading this account of Bill Logan and his community's work that the very presence of this switchboard, and others like it, saves lives. I wish that such a service had been there for me as I stumbled along through the process of 'coming out'. In the Australia that I lived within during the 1960s and 1970s heterosexuality was as taken for granted as breathing. Contemplating an existence outside of it was like contemplating living without breath.

I think of the coming out process as beginning well before an individual calls the Gay Switchboard. Even though I'm painfully aware of the way in which heterosexism smothers and tries to render them invisible, I still recognise a series of acts of resistance that I can trace back to my early adolescence and childhood. My path towards visibility as a lesbian involved daring to exist in a world that did not even have words for my existence.

I recognise that many of my gay friends struggle with homophobia and run the gamut of hate crimes which threaten their physical existence. As a woman, I have not been exposed to this degree of hate, even though I am always aware of the possibility. In my experience, sometimes an emphasis on homophobia can serve the purposes of heterosexism by rendering some of heterosexism's more subtle tactics invisible. Not that I don't think that homophobia needs to be exposed – it does. But somehow when homophobia is given all the attention, it can become OUR problem, something we have to deal with in therapy, when we come out and every day of our lives from that time on.

I think that heterosexism is an all-pervasive discourse and homophobia is one of its more obvious tactics, obvious because it results in hate crimes etc. which are becoming harder to cover up. Many straight people deny that they are homophobic but when it comes down to their assumption of heterosexual privilege, it becomes quite a different conversation. It is then that the subtleties of heterosexism start to be revealed. Sometimes it is not until they consider the fact that there is at least a ten per cent possibility that their child or children might be queer that heterosexual parents will look at their blindness and consider its impact on their children. I fantasise about my straight friends running a switchboard for straight people to help them deal with the impact of heterosexism on their families and their children.

Meanwhile, back in the real world, the existence of Gay Switchboard is a great symbol of resistance to heterosexism in all its forms, especially that of homophobia. I am so pleased to read about this account of narrative therapy in doing work with gay men who seek counsel over coming out. I know first-hand the power that these ideas have to liberate and to open up new ways of being and loving.

# 20

# A reflection

from

Christopher Behan

The idea of 'queer listening' in 'Weaving new stories over the phone' resonated for me. Bill Logan explains that the callers select the Gay Switchboard *because* the people answering the phone are gay and from this position the counsellors at the Switchboard actually listen in a particular way. These listening practices emphasise curiosity, especially around 'those elements that do not fit within a compulsory heterosexuality', and for the gaps in the narrative prescribed by heterosexual dominance. So, the grief and the heartache and the confusion the Switchboarders listen to may be seen as an expression of the caller's experience of the oppression within the dominant culture, and possibly as an expression of his hopes for a different sort of life.

**I will survive**

Bill links the history of the Gay Welfare Group and the Gay Switchboard to the post-Stonewall gay liberation movement of the late 1970s. Which takes me back in time. I can see myself at 16 in 1978 sitting in my room in Upstate New

York listening to Gloria Gaynor on the radio sing, 'I will survive. As long as I know how to love, I know I'll stay alive'. I was alone, didn't want to be gay, hated myself for it, pretended I was straight. Steeped in heterosexual dominance and isolated in a small town, I had no idea that that very song was an anthem of inspiration for gay men in discotheques in New York, San Francisco and around the world. In some ways that song saved me. Or maybe my hopes and dreams that things might be different were kept alive by disco songs like that. Sister Sledge's wisdom: 'We are family. I got all my sisters with me … have faith in you and the things you do. You won't go wrong. Oh, no. This is our family jewel.'

I didn't know about the drag queens who staged the Stonewall riots in 1969 to protest the raids on their neighbourhood bar. I didn't know about the hundreds of men and women who coalesced in the seventies and eighties to push the gay rights agenda forward – people like Bill Logan and Jerome and their collaborators on the Switchboard. In a sense, they made it possible for me to step into being seen and heard as a gay man when I finally came out in the early 1980s.

**Queer listening to Carl Rogers**

I find myself more excited by these connections than those Bill cited with Carl Rogers. Don't get me wrong; I have found Rogers' ideas helpful, especially in the level of technique, for example, reflecting back, reaching for feelings, etc. Rogers had a very positive, softening influence on the field of psychotherapy. Nonetheless, his ideas fit more into the humanist tradition with its notions of essentialism and other structuralist ideas of the self. The normalising gaze of humanism has done inestimable damage to gays, lesbians, bisexual and transgendered people. I prefer not to align with it.

I am not certain what others might say, but I find that the descr  on of the work on the Switchboard as 'Rogerian' does not sufficiently describe what I think is happening there. I think Bill's description of the work on the Switchboard as 'queer listening' is more rich and experience-near. Here he takes some of the ideas of narrative therapy and demonstrates their application in this particular context of talking with a gay man on a telephone hotline. This is 'copying that originates'. There are many lovely examples of this in Bill's paper:

- ***Exploring sparkling moments:*** I loved the part where Bill writes about how the Switchboarders get curious about the details of a unique outcome. 'We are interested in the colour of the other guy's hair and what he was wearing and the music that was playing.' Exploring these details accentuates the *momentousness* of the sparkling moment. I also find it refreshing to see how interested the Switchboarders are in the details of the sexual events that are judged by the callers to be preferred. Sex is a very important domain in the landscape of action! And sex is full of meaning to be explored in the landscape of consciousness too.

- ***Imagination:*** I appreciate that Bill would like to give more attention to 'the development of the future of caller's stories'. I think we could generate a wonderful list of questions that would help to tap into the imagination of a caller who is taking some of his first steps towards living openly as a gay man: 'Knowing what a wonderful time you had with Jeff last night, are you starting to wonder about a different kind of future for yourself?', 'Now that you are seeing how homophobia has interfered with your relationships with your family, what do you suppose you will want to do with it when you see it come up again?'

## Homophobia/heterosexual dominance

Bill's paper emphasised externalising homophobia as a way to 'separate the shame from the identity of the client by a manner of talking about the shame as an identity outside the person'. I too have found this to be a useful type of conversation to have with the gay men who consult me.

I realise that there is an ongoing debate about the use of terms of *heterosexual dominance* versus *homophobia* and about the fact that the two are often used interchangeably. Some feel that homophobia is too internalising a description of the problem, that it blames the victim. Laurence Carter illuminates the distinction between the two concepts in his essay 'Sunday Mowing' (1996). Speaking of homophobia:

> *Its connotation of rejection, active discrimination and violence are useful in maintaining a focus on the realities of living for many gay men ...*

*homophobia, directs the attention to the individual perpetrator of discrimination. Literally it describes these people as possessing fear of the same.*

It has been my experience that the idea of internalised homophobia has struck a chord for many of the men I have worked with over the years. Externalising homophobia helps to both emphasise the constitutive nature of culture which leads (some) gay men to fear and hate themselves and emphasise the agency of the person to live the kind of life he wishes. In the process of an externalising conversation, homophobia can be separated from the person, deconstructed as a cultural phenomenon and the person consulting me can be consulted about his position on it: 'So how does homophobia fit with the vision you have about the sort of life you would like to lead?'

On the other hand, Carter adds that:

*Heterosexual dominance is marked by a curiosity to comprehend the cultural context of the injustice. It is a way of challenging the supported values and imperatives that maintain the injustice.*

Speaking in terms of heterosexual dominance highlights the privileged position of heterosexuals and inherent social injustice. So I frequently talk with my clients in externalising the effects of heterosexual dominance. I think this makes it even clearer that the problems that many of the men who consult me experience (self-hatred, depression, substance abuse, suicidality) are the outcome of a social process.

Personally I have found both concepts helpful in my work. Laurence also comes to the conclusion that the ideas are not in any way mutually exclusive:

*The understandings and experiences that lead people to use one term or other term are reinforcing of each other, and reflect varying views on the same concern and challenge for change.*

**Being heard**

Also, I find myself fascinated with the idea of 'queer listening', as a special kind of listening within narrative therapy. Much of my work in assisting gay men in breaking free from the negative effects of heterosexual dominance and homophobia has had more to do with being *seen*. Often we are co-authoring preferred stories that work with metaphors about becoming visible. Given Bill's experience as a telephone counsellor, it makes sense that listening and being heard might be emphasised. I have also found the metaphor of finding one's own voice to be a useful way to frame the alternative narrative.

For so many gay men living in the closet, no-one has been listening, or no-one wants to hear about 'the love that dare not speak its name', least of all other men. What I think I see in the Gay Switchboard's group is men transforming men's culture, especially some of its most problematic aspects – homophobia, intolerance of alternative ways of expressing 'maleness', oppression of those who do not conform to norms, and more. I am convinced that as men we are accountable to the rest of society to change men's ways of being that continue to perpetrate social injustice. I admire the way that Bill and his friends at the Gay Switchboard are making it happen.

If identities are constituted within communities, it seems to me that the Gay Switchboard is a site of resistance to the taken-for-granted practices of heterosexual dominance. The Switchboard provides access to alternative ways of thinking and being in the world that are more free from heterosexual dominance. It seems to me that for some it is literally a gateway to a new life where being loved by another man is honoured, where one's sexuality is not considered shameful or dangerous, and where connection in a community of other gay men is possible.

# 21

# A reflection

from

Claire Ralfs

## Queer Listening

Upon reading Bill's paper, I have really enjoyed trying to think through my beliefs about 'queer listening'. This has been a great process and one for which I have Bill and his community to thank.

In thinking through taking on a gay or lesbian identity, because of the influences of heterosexual dominance and other factors, there are often dilemmas and difficulties to be faced as well as things to celebrate. It seems to me that queer listening involves respecting the diversity of people's actual experiences of this process. One hope I would have is that we as workers could enable people to acknowledge the diversity and complexities of their experiences in relation to their sexuality. For me, this involves something more than listening for things that are good about being gay or lesbian, or the positive aspects of coming out. It is also something quite different than inviting people into claiming an identity of gay or lesbian. For lots of reasons, it can be problematic to invite people who are just starting to make statements about their sexuality and about their sexual identities, into needing to make choices between heterosexual or homosexual identities.

As Bill's paper invited me to think about this, I was reminded of a young woman who came and talked with me when I was working at Family Planning. She was in a relationship at that time with a lesbian woman who very much wanted her to come out and be in a particular way as a lesbian. This particular way did not fit for her at that time. Since then, this young woman now lives what I would call a fairly lesbian-identified life, but at that point in time she was finding it very unhelpful to think that she had to make a choice between heterosexual identity on the one hand and a particular lesbian identity on the other. Trying to make choices between absolutes was creating dilemmas for her.

It seems to me that it is the absolutes imposed by heterosexual dominance that create much of the oppression for our relationships. While the temptation to impose an alternative identity is strong, creating an understanding of relationships and sexual identities that are not necessarily fixed is far more exciting. Finding ways to stand up to the absolutes for those newly seeking to explore alternative ways of being is an important foundation for the queer movement. The whole issue of bisexuality is relevant here. In my opinion making people choose an identity holds us back from exploring the many ways all of us – gay, lesbian, bisexual, heterosexual, undecided – can challenge the dominance of heterosexuality.

Some of the dilemmas which many people experience relate to the fact that the visible identities of 'gay' or 'lesbian' are usually those defined in relation to the perspectives of first-world gay and lesbian people who live in cities, and who are often fairly affluent. Many people who are trying to come terms with same-sex desire do not live in cities, are not affluent, do not come from white western cultural backgrounds and do not identify themselves as gay or lesbian. I recall a recent study from Victoria which describes men in rural Australian contexts who regularly enjoy sexual contact with other men but who don't identify as gay in any way. What I understand this research is saying is that these are valid choices made by people in their lives and it does not make sense to interpret their actions through the lens of an inner-city gay or lesbian worldview. Similarly, looking at cross-cultural situations, living out lesbian or gay relationships if you are from a Macedonian community or an Aboriginal community, is very different than those ways of living that are promoted within a lot of the core identified gay and lesbian communities. This means that lesbians and gay men from non-western cultural communities often feel as if they are forced to choose between their cultural communities and the gay and lesbian community. I would hope that as we develop better skills in queer listening that we will become more aware of the effects of invitations to choose between absolute identities of either gay/lesbian or heterosexual.

Queer listening, then, rather than inviting people into particular identities, can involve instead closely listening for what people want. The young woman I described before wanted opportunities to mix with alternative communities but to not have to name herself. So we talked about ways to make this possible. Having a time in which she did not have to state an identity was something that she particularly wanted.

Noticing the directions in which people want to be taking their lives, and being open to these directions rather than interpreting them, seems important. As Bill describes, creating conversational contexts in which people can separate themselves from the effects of homophobia is invaluable. I am interested in how, throughout this process, we can ensure that the people we are talking with are in charge of interpreting the meanings of events in their lives and the directions in which they wish to move. If someone does not wish to come out at a particular time or in a particular way, this may not be due to the effects of homophobia, but instead to particular wishes they have for their lives in their own contexts. Queer listening needs to not only externalise homophobia but also enable people to make their own meaning out of their lives and sexualities.

Queer listening may also involve eliciting ways in which people are looking for and finding support to take the steps that they want to take. We might explore how this support could be enhanced, for example through listening groups, as Bill describes.

I was interested in Bill's explorations of sparkling moments. These explorations seem very important. Sparkling moments that I would be interested in listening for might include the connections that people have with others who are validating their preferred relationship structures. We can listen for people and for moments that have assisted the person to live out and live with the complexities of their lives, and we can explore ways in which these connections, and the meanings of these connections, can be enriched.

As people who have lived outside the conventional relationship structures of the culture, we have had at times a fierceness at claiming alternative identities. There is sometimes a great sense of relief in claiming identities that are clearly not heterosexual. Having support to do so can be crucial. However, if we embrace these identities as absolutes, we can find we become limited in our ability to enjoy the exciting and challenging diversity of people's loves and lives. In terms of working with people who are still in the early process of making their identities, I am interested in how we can take extra special care in remaining fully appreciative of the complexities of the process and not fall into the trap of imposing gay or lesbian absolutes. In this way we can continue to evolve our skills in queer listening.

# 22

# A reflection

from

Patrick O'Leary

## An invitation into complexities

I very much enjoyed reading Bill's paper and hearing about the work that he and his community are doing to address the effects of homophobia in the lives of the men who ring Gay Switchboard. As a heterosexual man who works with men and young men whose lives have been affected by sexual abuse, I find the influence of homophobia in men's lives is becoming increasingly apparent and important to me.

In my conversations with young men, I regularly hear of the ways in which homophobia is used to intimidate them, and how it influences their considerations of choice in their sexual lives. This seems true for young men regardless of how they might be identifying in relation to their sexual orientation. Of course for young men who identify as gay, bisexual, transgender, queer, or are identified by others as such, there are the effects of discrimination and often violence to contend with as well.

For men who have had experiences of child sexual abuse from other men – and it is important to clarify that this abuse is mostly perpetrated by men who are living heterosexual lives – homophobia can have particularly complex and destructive effects. Sometimes homophobia, when linked with an abusive same-sex experience, can invite men into thinking that any same-sex feeling, desire or action that they have must in some way be linked to the abuse. For men who have experienced abuse and who also experience same-sex desire, this can really encourage destructive self-blame. Homophobia can also invite people into thinking that the abusive experiences they suffered were terrible because the acts involved same-sex sex and this can make invisible the power dynamics that made the abuse what it was.

In my experience, these complexities mean that it is really important in a counselling situation to be allowing room for men and young men to define their sexuality and sexual identity in whatever way is appropriate for them. I have found it helpful to invite those who consult with me to be open to the idea that sexuality and sexual identity is not fixed, and how for many men and women it can and does change throughout life and in different contexts.

In having conversations with men who have experienced same-sex abuse, I have found it very important to invite conversations that allow men to articulate and name their experiences as abuses of power. Considering the effects of power in situations of abuse makes it clear that entering into these sexual acts was not a choice that they were making. What can also be significant is to be able to share some of the sorts of conversations that I've had with other men about the confusion that sexual abuse can bring, so that no man has to feel alone with confusion around these issues.

One of the other things I find relevant in these conversations is to contextualise them in relation to dominant constructions of masculinity. I try to make clear that talking openly with another man about intimate experiences requires some skills and qualities as it is an act that challenges dominant constructions of masculinity. To enter into these conversations often indicates hopes and dreams about different ways that life could be for a man, and we can explore these in therapy. I am also careful to contextualise the fact that there are few places where it is 'safe' or wise to be talking with other men about same-sex desire, and that sometimes not talking about these things has been a sign of good judgement. I try to find ways to make it clear that I am comfortable and willing to talk about same-sex attraction and sexuality – not only in relation to acts of abuse, but also as choices in the realm of delight, love and hope.

One of the real hopes I had while reading Bill's article was thinking how it may inspire others, particularly those like myself within the heterosexual community, to think about our responsibilities in addressing homophobia. I was reminded of the article 'Questioning sexuality' by Mark Trudinger, Cameron Boyd and Peter Melrose (1998), and I am very interested in considering this questioning further.

If homophobia was not something that young men had to contend with in relation to dealing with the effects of sexual abuse, I believe it would be much less intimidating for young men to speak out about abuse. And if it was less intimidating for young men to speak out about abuse, it would make a difference for how long men would have to carry around the effects of the abuse in their lives. These ideas are really understandings that have come from my conversations with men who have spoken about the ways in which homophobia was used to intimidate them into silence. I remember one man saying to me, 'If homophobia wasn't around, it would make it a lot harder for men that abuse to get away with it'. This was a really important thought for this man. The men who had abused him were heterosexual men and he believed that if they had not had homophobia as an ally in secrecy, his life would have been far less affected by sexual abuse.

If homophobia was less present in our culture, I think we might also be able to get clearer about what it is that constitutes sexual abuse. Perhaps if the broader community addressed homophobia, it would also make it easier to delineate between abusive same-sex experiences, coercive same-sex experiences, confusing but kind of mutually muddily same-sex experiences, consenting and delightful same-sex experiences, transformative same-sex experiences etc. etc. With homophobia reduced, we'd be able to develop richer descriptions of sex, both heterosexual and homosexual. I think this would make it easier for all of us to have a language to better describe our experiences.

In working with men and young men who are trying to come to terms with the effects of sexual abuse, and who are trying to construct a sexual identity that fits for them, my concern is how to ensure that they have the space, the language, the tools and the time to do this in their own way. Some may identify strongly as gay, bisexual, transgender or heterosexual. Others may be finding their way between or through all these different understandings.

Somehow tied up with homophobia is the idea that if you as a man have a forced same-sex experience, this will necessarily change your sexual identity –

that somehow experiencing coerced same-sex means that you are gay. This can become further complicated if men have experienced any physiological arousal from the experience. Because of these societal beliefs, it seems all the more important that in a counselling situation men can find their own way – be that to embrace a homosexual, heterosexual or other sexual identity.

Finally, there are also complexities present in relation to exploring sparkling sexual moments. I believe that when asking men about their first same-sex sexual experiences, it is important to recognise that these may not necessarily have been sparkling at all. They may have occurred in a context of shame, or a context of tentativeness, or even coercion. Or, their first sexual experiences may not have been sparkling at the time, but have come to be seen as sparkling in hindsight – that they were first steps towards a preferred identity. Alternatively the reverse could be true, there have been incidences in my life which at the time I saw as sparkling but later came to understand differently.

So in conversations about these matters, I am interested in hearing people's own judgements about what have been sparkling moments in their lives in relation to their sexual identity. These may or may not be their early sexual experiences, whether the person identifies as heterosexual, homosexual, bisexual, transgender or queer.

Sparkling moments in relation to sexual identity might not even relate to specific sexual acts; instead they may involve ways of relating that are associated with a certain sexual orientation. I think these explorations can lead to rich conversations.

I am interested in checking out whether an event really is a sparkling moment, by asking questions like: 'Would you see this as a sparkling moment in your stands against homophobia?', or 'Would you see this as a beginning point in your stand against homophobia?'. Or perhaps a predictive question such as, 'In five years' time, how do you think you'd see this moment?' In relation to people's early sexual experiences, be they same-sex or different-sex experiences, I'd be interested in leaving some space for movement in interpretation of the events. The influences of homophobia, of puritan attitudes towards sexuality in our culture, and the incidence of sexual abuse mean that issues of sexuality and sexual identity have a complexity that we as counsellors need to acknowledge and work with. I think Bill's paper is a great invitation into considering these complexities and finding ways for us all to address the many differing effects of homophobia.

# 23

# *Reflections on reflections*

from

*Bill Logan*

I found the comments on my paper inspiring, stimulating and helpful – and some of the lines of discussion just leave me in unresolved thought. I found Claire Ralfs' injunction to respect the fluidity always possible in sexual life salutary. It is always of great sustenance to me to hear personal stories like Christopher Behan and Zoy Kazan, who talk of transcending the isolation and loneliness to the point of wordlessness for our experiences – and coming out! Accounts of working with people who've been sexually abused always move me, and somehow abusive homosexual acts as talked of by Patrick O'Leary have their special twist for me.

The Gay Switchboard has a tradition, but it is – always, I hope – in a process of change. This paper itself, in an earlier version, was circulated as a reflection for the Switchboard on its work, and thereby contributed to the changes going on in the current phase of its history. And perhaps the reflections on the paper published here will further contribute to the process.

Christopher's comments on Rogerianism might well engage Switchboarders. While lots of our formal training sessions have for many years been in the vocabulary of Rogerianism, it is my impression that, in Christopher's words 'this does not sufficiently describe what ... is happening here'. In practice something else far more interesting and helpful has been going on.

I think Christopher and Zoy points to a danger that might flow from the paper if it were to lead to fixing on homophobia as the only problem to be externalised for people in the process of coming out. Of course in practice words for many of the specific externalised problems arise out of the life and talk of the caller – often 'shame', 'fear', and so on. We introduce new concepts carefully, and we do so for the purpose of setting these specific 'personal' problems in their social context, and in order to deconstruct the dominant culture which shapes that context. In the Switchboard tradition, we have found that 'homophobia' serves well as a broad term for the beginning of that process, and that it can often be given much of the content of 'heterosexual dominance' and 'heterosexism' (and bigotry, , family expectations, anti-gay prejudice, heterosexism, and so on). But just as the peoples of the Arctic need many different words for 'snow', so queer people need a sophisticated vocabulary to describe an alien cultural environment.

The intersection of sexual abuse and homophobia discussed by Patrick seems an enormously important field, and although a bit outside the scope of the paper as originally conceived, it's a useful topic because it presents itself so often in this kind of work. Abuse shrouded by secrecy is doubly pernicious and, as Patrick shows, the secrecy bred by homophobia compounds the distresses and confusions facing so many men.

This paper was originally written for other members of the Gay Switchboard. If I had been thinking about how these stories might be read by non-gay readers, I wonder if I would have written differently about the ways in which we story the detail of those sexual experiences callers' have which escape the problem-saturated story. Some non-gay readers and perhaps some gay readers might wish I had. But no! The problem the dominant culture has with queerness is that it involves SEX between people of the same gender. There is a lot more to being gay than sex, but it is the sex which problematises it – for the dominant culture and therefore for the emergent gay or bisexual person.

# PART SIX

# *Bisexual experience*

These three diverse papers attempt to articulate the experience, politics and implications of bisexuality.

# 24

# Sometimes bisexuality is...

by

David Denborough

Sometimes bisexual identity is an honouring of what has been. It stands firmly and cries out 'we loved each other, it existed, I must not let that history fade. I must tell and retell the existence of that love, it was/is so much a part of me and my life.'

In some situations bisexual identity visits people's lives for a short time.

In other situations it flows through people's spirits forever and is a life-long way of living and understanding life.

Sometimes bisexual identity is a possibility.

Sometimes bisexuality is a uncomplicated delight in bodies of different shapes and sizes.

Sometimes bisexual identity asks to be accepted, that it's just like everyone else, please let us in.

Other times bisexual identity dances and spins, sings out 'we're not like everyone else', come and play over here if you like.

Sometimes bisexuality is a movement, a pulse, creating space for people to move with greater ease and fluidity.

Sometimes bisexuality can be loud, brash and try to barge into sacred spaces carefully carved out over decades.

Sometimes bisexuality is an intellectual argument, other times it's a question mark.

Sometimes bisexuality is a passion which refuses to be confined.

Sometimes bisexuality is a place where people meet and talk. A place that once didn't exist. A place that has been created due to those who have lived lives off the straight and narrow – and those who have loved and supported them along the way.

Other times bisexuality is a language still in construction. New letters, words and syllables evolving each day.

Sometimes harassment, condescension, assumption and judgement follow bisexuality around.

But joy, curiosity, challenge and delight are its favourite companions. Bisexuality can be cheeky!

# 25

# Beyond happy endings

## Identity politics, bisexuality, narrative

by

Frann Michel

In 1978, I was a sixteen-year-old college freshman in New York City. Bisexual chic had been discovered by *Time & Newsweek* four years earlier, Elton John was bisexual, Kate Millet was bisexual, and Margaret Mead had said in *Redbook* that maybe everyone was. To point to such circumstances is to suggest that they are relevant, that they in some way explain the outcome of the anecdote. But this is an artefact of narrative strategy, a retrospective foregrounding of events that may not at the time have seemed important. The end of the story gives meaning to the details, tells the teller which details matter, offers the satisfaction of closure. If endings don't always define stories, they nonetheless help define their genres. Renaissance and classical tragedies, for instance, end in death; comedies end in marriage. Detective stories end in resolution of the enigma, the answer to who done it. Conversion narratives explain how I came to be as I am, how I came to Grace or Truth. Sexual identity narratives, coming out stories, are much like conversion narratives. And the stories that we read influence the stories we can tell. The sense we make of fictions reflects the sense we make of our lives.

Identity as static category may tell us what our history has made us, but not what we might make of our history. Describing the past so as to explain the present creates closure, an end or aim, both terminus and goal. But some goals are more valued than others. The question of bisexual identity has been particularly vexed; a generation of bisexual feminist women were accused by other feminists of disloyalty for not identifying as lesbian. That this has changed is largely due to the work of bisexual activists, but it is also due to a growing scepticism about identity itself. How can one find a stable and satisfactory position within an unsatisfactory social system? Bisexual identity as a viable and visible position in queer politics has emerged concurrently with a critique of identity politics. Whether as cause or effect of this paradox, bisexuality has become a focus for alternative understandings of identity as narrative.

Some of the political scepticism about identity derives from a historicising of its categories. According to Michel Foucault, 'sexuality' was invented some time in the 18th century in Europe. The Oxford English Dictionary locates the term's emergence at 1800, though scholars disagree about exactly when the concept developed. The important point, however, is that it is an historical development, and is a culturally-specific concept, rather than an essential something that is always and everywhere the same. In *The History of Sexuality* (volume one), Foucault traces a shift in the way the Catholic church structured confession, from asking about acts to asking about desires. The invention of sexuality does not mean that prior to 1800 (or whenever) people did not do things we can recognise as engaging in sexual acts or feeling sexual desires, nor does it mean that they did not value them. The point is that they did not think of these desires and acts in the same way as central to their identities. Foucault traces a shift from acts to identities, for example, from sodomy (a kind of behaviour) to homosexuals (a kind of person). He links this to a broader shift in structures of power, from a feudal 'right of death' in which the king could kill his subjects, to a 'power over life' in which control is more pervasive. Public execution, for instance, was replaced by incarceration and surveillance. In *Discipline and Punish*, Foucault discusses Jeremy Bentham's design for the panopticon, a prison in which every cell would be visible to guards; not knowing when they might be observed, prisoners would learn to discipline themselves.

In this argument, sexual identities are points of social control, of subjectification, of making subjects who are docile. The internal self-scrutiny entailed in making sure one is 'normal' or in cataloguing one's deviance is part of the larger internalisation of controls that assure order in developed societies. The energy devoted to self-monitoring may be diverted from challenges to the existing political and economic structures. It may even make envisioning such challenges more difficult. As Louis Althusser notes, in responding to a call, a name, the subject implicitly accepts the linguistic and social structure from which the call or name emerges. Because we answer to the names our society makes available, the violent imposition of external order is less necessary.

**Identity politics**

But sexual identities can also be points of resistance, subversion, through what Foucault calls reverse discourses. A reverse discourse develops when people claim for themselves the terms that have been imposed on them by others. Turning externally decreed labels into self-chosen names, this reversal can change the top-down ordering of passive populations into the means for organising grassroots activism. Thus subject categories that were developed as taxonomising tools of control can be turned around, revalued, used as tools of resistance though reverse discourse. In that sense, the whole notion of gay liberation or gay rights is a reverse discourse, a claiming of an imposed identity in order to exercise agency, a claiming of agency in regard to such a category. A more local example would be the revaluing of words like 'queer', claiming it as a positive term. The more popular understanding of such reverse discourses in recent history is in terms of identity politics. Identity politics is the idea that one's political beliefs and actions will come out of one's identity. It grew in part out of reaction to the New Left analyses which privileged class and economic structures over structures of race, gender, sexuality. Hence, it also refers to politics focused on such social or identity issues. Identity politics developed in the context of the 1960s and 1970s liberation struggles: Black people worked for Black power, women worked for women's liberation, and gay people worked for gay liberation.

Identity politics has sometimes been critiqued for being too narrowly focused. In this pejorative sense, 'identity politics' tends to refer to approaches which neglect, in particular, economic analysis, and, in general, any of the identity components by which the practitioners in question are privileged rather than oppressed. Thus, the identity politics of straight white women might attend to gender but neglect race and sexuality. A related critique of identity politics is that it can lead to what is sometimes described as 'victim politics', in which the experience of victimisation or oppression is grounds for articulation of grievances and appeal for redress, but in which the movement of articulation is not seen as the beginning of transformation of the oppressed identity. In 'La Guera', Cherrie Moraga writes:

> *Do we merely struggle with the 'ism' that's sitting on top of our own heads? The answer is: yes, I think first we do; and we must do so thoroughly and deeply. But to fail to move out from there will only isolate us in our own oppression – will only insulate, rather than radicalize us.* (p.29).

That is, the categories of identity politics cannot be simply dispensed with, since they have generated important transformations of a politics based on economic critique. Identity politics, in some of its uses, functions as a useful starting place. But it needs to be transcended: the Combahee River Collective, in their classic statement on identity politics, note that they began with antiracist and antisexist politics, but *as we developed politically we addressed ourselves to hetero-sexism and economic oppression under capitalism* (p.212).

Identity politics has also been critiqued for suggesting that being part of an oppressed group will necessarily lead to radical analysis of that oppression. One source of the misconception that identity politics is necessarily the root of radical politics, and the most significant critique of identity politics, lies in the question of what 'identity' is. The first meaning of 'identity' in the Oxford English Dictionary is *The quality or condition of being the same in substance, composition, nature, properties, or in particular qualities under consideration; absolute or essential sameness; oneness.* The second is *The sameness of a person or thing at all times or in all circumstances; the condition or fact that a person or thing is itself and not something else; individuality, personality.* The definition used generally in the notion of identity politics seems to combine these two meanings. But both of these notions of identity have been critiqued. The idea that there is an absolute or essential sameness in the particular quality of being, say, African-American, or female, is belied not only by the evident political differences between people of the 'same' race or gender, but also by the problem of pinning down precisely what that quality might be. In the case of gender, for instance, neither chromosomes, nor genitals, nor any other feature provides a clear, consistent, dividing line between different genders. Women-only groups have faced conflicts over accepting transsexual women, and the work of transgendered and intersexual activists has further made visible the complexity of constructions of gender. In addition, as feminists of colour pointed out about the white women's movement, for instance, the term 'woman' was actually used to refer to white women – and, indeed, to straight, middle-class white women – a subset of the category as conventionally understood. Race and gender are not essential categories but social ones. Moreover, the idea that an individual person is always the same at all times and in all circumstances is equally problematic.

**Bisexual politics**

Bisexual politics has emerged in the face of this scepticism about organising around identity categories. Like other identities, bisexual identity is not something that develops simply out of an individual's need, but is instead a function of power and a consequence of history. The earliest meaning of 'bisexual' offered in the Oxford English Dictionary refers to the inclusion of both sexes in a single individual: what might more commonly be called androgyny, hermaphroditism, or transgender. As late as the 1971 edition this was the only definition listed, though sexologists and psychoanalysts by the turn of the century were using the term to refer to desire for both sexes. But this meaning of the term (focusing on desire, rather than anatomy) was not popularly disseminated until the 1970s, after the Stonewall rebellion and the rise of gay liberation movements. While bisexual behaviour surely existed earlier, it could not become a focus of identity, a term of self-identification, until the word became available. To project bisexual identity onto figures in the past who lived in periods before the term was in use or before it was used as an identity-concept, or who live in places where it isn't an identity-concept, is to engage in an anachronistic or culturally imperialist projection.

Even after 'bisexual' became available as a term of self-description, its meaning remained contentious. Newly visible bisexuals were derided as promiscuous, indecisive, and untrustworthy. Lesbian feminist theory of the 1970s came to equate political commitment to women with sexual commitment to women, and both with a turning away from men. Even as the term became more familiar as a possible identity, then, feminist women were pressured not only by the heterosexism of straight society, but also by lesbian feminist critiques of that heterosexism to choose sides. One couldn't, in some views, be a feminist and still have sex with men. Adrienne Rich, in her landmark 1981 essay 'Compulsory Heterosexuality and Lesbian Existence', characterised bisexuality as 'a liberal leap across the tasks and struggles of here and now'. Thus even those who endorsed identity politics criticised the identity bisexual.

Bisexual activists have responded to these critiques not only with specific rebuttals, but also, and more significantly, with explorations of the ways bisexuality can help reconceptualise identity. The difficulty of pinning down a definition of bisexuality points to the difficulty of pinning down a definition of any sexual subjectivity. Bisexuality is the capacity to feel sexual attraction to people of more than one gender, or the experience of being sexual with people of more than one gender (whether concurrently or serially), or the identification of oneself as bisexual on the basis of such attraction or experience. These definitions may overlap or conflict. That is, one might feel sexual attraction to people of more than one gender and have sexual experiences with people of more than one gender, and yet identify as straight or gay on the basis of stronger attraction to one gender or the other, or on the basis of social affiliations or political beliefs. Or, one might identify as bisexual without having had any sexual experiences, or having had sexual experiences with people of only one gender. One might identify as bisexual without feeling any sexual attractions at all. And so on. That is, the term is adopted for varied reasons and motives, to describe various configurations of sexual subjectivity. While this is also true of other sexual identities, they are less often called upon to define themselves.

The extravagant charges against bisexuality (that it doesn't exist, for instance) have perhaps led to some of the comparably extravagant claims by defenders of bisexuality (that everyone is bisexual, for example). Some have seen in bisexuality's capacity to problematise categories of identity a revolutionary potential. For psychologist Beth Firestein (1996), the blurring of 'distinctions between apparently different sexual orientations' undermines both the categories and the hierarchical relation between them, so that 'discrimination becomes impossible' (p.283). But such utopian claims do seem open to Rich's charge of leaping over the problems of the present. Even without claiming the revolution has been won, however, we may note that bisexuality has been understood as standing for a variety of challenges to the current hetero/sexist normative scheme, as pointing (despite its prefix) beyond binary organisations of gender and sexuality. Firestein sees it as pointing toward a LesBiGay/Transgender affirmative paradigm which recognises that the many labels indicating sexual identity:

> *... do not denote entirely discrete populations, but rather represent the self-identification of individuals whose feelings and experiences contain substantial overlap and whose identification choices are influenced as much by sociopolitical considerations and the heterosexism of the broader society as by reference to their actual sexual behaviour and feelings.* (p.281)

The sociopolitical considerations shaping sexual self-identification might include race, class, gender, and other axes of social organisation. In particular, a number of writers, including June Jordan (1994), Lani Ka'ahumanu (1995), and many of the contributors to the anthology *Plural Desires*, have noted an analogy between multiracial and bisexual identities and politics. June Jordan writes in 'A new politics of sexuality':

> *I do believe that the analogy for bisexuality is a multicultural, multi-ethnic, multiracial world view. Bisexuality follows from such a perspective and leads to it as well.* (p.192)

Jordan points to the ways that people of multiracial backgrounds have multiple heritages to honour; in this sense the comparison is to multiple communities: bisexual and multiracial people have multiple traditions. Jordan emphasises the importance of valuing complexity. These identities foreground in a way the limitations of identity politics, since one cannot locate identity in a single community. Even queer people of colour who do not specifically identify as multiracial may have similar experiences. For instance, Indigo Som (1995) discusses Asian identity as disrupting the conventional racial binary of black/white. Like bisexuality, then, attention to racial and ethnic positionings other than black or white can add to the complexity of the cultural map. Brenda

Marie Blasingame (1992) suggests that bisexual behaviour is common in communities of colour, and that given the racism of (white) lesbian/gay communities, and the homophobia of (straight) black communities, some black queer people may have relationships in both worlds. Thus bisexuality may be a strategy for moving between communities, or a manifestation of participation in multiple communities. Thus the analogies between bisexual and multiracial politics are not purely theoretical, but rather signs of material overlap; they offer clues to coalition-building and to the development of richer and more complex communities, beyond narrowly defined identities.

Ka'ahumanu writes in 'It ain't over 'till the bisexual speaks':

> *Like multiculturalism, / mixed heritage and bi-racial relationships, / both the bisexual and transgender movements / expose and politicise the middle ground.* (p.64)

Both Jordan and Ka'ahumanu characterise bisexuality as politicising the middle ground (or what Jordan calls the 'so-called middle ground' [p.193]). Bisexuality is thus characterised in spatial terms, though both Jordan and Ka'ahumanu would reject the spatially similar but pejorative notion of 'fence-sitting'. The notion that the middle ground is not (yet) politicised suggests a model of politics as binary, as war by other means, as a dualistic struggle. The idea of politicising this territory means constructing another model of politics. Ka'ahumanu suggests that bisexual and transgender movements show:

> *... there is no separation,/that each and everyone of us/is part of a fluid social, sexual, and gender dynamic. // Each signals a change, a fundamental change / in the way our society is organized.* (p.64)

This signal points not to an accomplishment but to an agenda, a change in the making.

Jordan suggests that:

> *Bisexuality invalidates either/or formulation, either/or analysis. Bisexuality means I am free and I am as likely to want and to love a woman as I am likely to want and love a man, and what about that? Isn't that what freedom implies? If you are free, you are not predictable and you are not controllable.* (p.193)

Of course, there is a polemical dimension to these writings. The equation of bisexuality with freedom, for instance, or at least with a declaration of freedom, emerges as a response to specific restrictions, but asserts a more general liberation that it is also calling for as:

> ... *a unifying, 1990s mandate for revolutionary Americans planning to make it into the twenty-first century on the basis of the heart, on the basis of an honest human body, consecrated to every struggle for justice, every struggle for equality, every struggle for freedom.* (p.193)

These are the concluding words of Jordan's essay, first delivered as a lecture, and they have a rhetorical force meant to mobilise audience energies toward struggles for justice, equality, and freedom. Thus, though bisexuality is asserted as an already available freedom, it also functions as a rhetorical tool in the struggle to achieve a projected freedom. The existence anywhere of bisexuality cannot plausibly be said to invalidate either/or analysis everywhere, but it can function as a tool, a reminder to problematise either/or analysis, and a mode of thinking through that questioning of binary formulations. The analogies asserted between bisexual and multiracial movements can function to call forth what they are asserting is already present. The visibility of people who are neither black nor white can (should) undermine, forestall simplistic thinking about not only race but also about other identity categories. Jordan comments that:

> ... *the keenly positive, politicizing significance of bisexual affirmation* is its capacity *to insist upon the equal validity of all the components of social/sexual complexity.* (p.193)

**Narrative possibilities**

To explicate this complexity, and as another response to the inadequacy of terms or labels, some bisexual theorists suggest emphasising narrative. Legal theorist Ruth Colker, in her book *Hybrid: Bisexuals, multiracials, and other misfits under American law* (1996) suggests that one way to make more visible the individuals who lie between legally recognised categories is:

> *to embrace individualised storytelling rather than categories such as 'bisexual' ... Categories suggest stasis whereas storytelling reflects our changing life experiences.* (p.19)

Bisexuality is particularly likely to lead to such a move because, while categories of homosexual and heterosexual (and their variants) give the illusion of structures, bisexuality can only be visually framed with images of three people. Representation of serial bisexuality requires narrative.

Thus bisexual identity has been repeatedly theorised in relation to narrative, and indeed as narrative (Garber 1995, p.87). Literary scholar Marjorie Garber emphasises bisexuality as a way of making sense of a life story that includes same-sex and other-sex desires. In one sense, this understanding of bisexuality is a way of preserving a coherent identity through change and fluidity. Paradoxically, bisexual identity as such can become a tool to construct coherence. There might be fluidity in location in relation to acts and communities, without having to engage a parallel fluidity of terminology. There is a paradox or tension between designating a particular identity as bisexual and wanting to emphasise bisexuality as fluidity or as standing for potential and change, between the stability of 'identity' and the flexibility signalled by 'bisexuality'. Garber unites these by emphasising varieties of experience over the course of a life. This makes of identity something that does not exist only in acts, behaviours, or community locations at a particular moment. It resides rather in memory and desire. But this is presumably true in a sense of any identity – bisexuality is just one that makes it more visible than others.

Like lesbian and gay theorising, bisexual writings have begun with an emphasis on coming-out stories and other personal narratives, but the structure of those narratives differs considerably. Lesbian coming-out stories gain their meaning from the end of the story. As literary critic Biddy Martin (1988) has noted, the contributions to collections like *The Coming Out Stories, The New Lesbians*, and *The Lesbian Path* offer narratives constructed through cultural feminist analyses that locate 'the key to opposing male supremacy' in 'withdrawal from men, now named lesbianism' (p.86). Emphasising woman-identification as the authenticating unity of sexuality, subjectivity, and political stance, these narratives offer a linear progression from confusion or lies to a return to an essential, true self and desire, *grounding identity and political unity in moral right and truth* (p.89). Thus the ending of the story – the arrival at lesbian identity – shapes the meaning of what has come before. Garber describes such stories as 'conversion narratives' (p.347), and notes:

> [w]*e begin with the 'end' of the story, and retell it so that it 'comes out right', producing, as if inevitably from the materials of a life, the person we (think we) are now.* (p.324)

Such essentialising narratives postulate a purely constative mode, one that obscures the extent to which discourse constructs rather than merely reflects the truth of experience and identity. Thus in both the hetero and lesbian versions of. such narratives, whom one ends up with indicates what one's sexuality really is.

Lesbian narratives of bisexuality have had a similar structure, in which the monosexual ending constructs the meaning of what has come before. The Gay Revolution Party Women's Caucus's 1971 essay, 'Realesbians and Politicalesbians', for instance, comments:

> *The claim to bisexuality is commonly heard within the movement, and while bisexuality is not physiologically impossible, the term cannot be used to characterize a stable socio-sexual orientation. Because no heterosexual relationship is free of power politics and other masculine mystifications, women who assert that they are bisexual retain their definition by men and the social advantages accruing from this. Bisexuality is a transitional stage, a middle ground, through which women pass from oppressive relationships to those of equality and mutuality. It is a struggle with privilege and fear, and not all women come through it to their sisters on the other side.* (pp.179-180)

In the intervening years lesbian relationships have been somewhat demystified, and can no longer be so easily romanticised. Relationships between women can no longer be assumed to be free of power politics and necessarily characterised by equality and mutuality, for instance. Yet the presentation of bisexuality formulated here still has a good deal of currency. Many lesbian feminists still read bisexuality as complicity with the institution of heterosexuality and a rejection or denial of the critique of that institution. In this account, bisexuality is necessarily part of a larger narrative, and indeed it manifests the disequilibrium characteristic of narrative. Construing bisexuality as an unstable transitional stage on the way to the telos of lesbian identification frames it as part of a conventionalised, linear, lesbian coming-out narrative.

This mode of storytelling and of reading, in which endings give meaning to what has come before, has played a central role in western culture, as Frank Kermode argues in *The Sense of an Ending* (1966). But clearly it interferes with reading bisexuality, and thus with the models for narrating a bisexual story. Film theorist Maria Pramaggiore notes that in classical cinema:

> *romantic coupling and temporal closure are related narrative structures ... Coupling signifies completion, wholeness, and stasis and usually suggests a diachronically stable object choice*;

and she suggests that such chronological narrative structures may be less compatible with:

> *... bisexual reading strategies, which focus on the episodic quality of a nonteleological temporal continuum across which a number of sexual acts, desires, and identities might be expressed.* (1996, p.277)

In an analysis of lesbian readings of classical Hollywood films such as *Morocco* and *Queen Christina*, film critic Judith Mayne (1991) notes a conflict between the potentially lesbian spectacle offered by particular scenes, and the narrative structures of the films, which are directed toward heterosexual closure. Mayne argues for a 'both/and' reading of the conflict between narrative and spectacle as fundamentally ironic, and connects this reading process with a bisexuality that provokes a 'crisis in representation' (pp.117, 131). Mayne emphasises the importance of keeping *these two dynamics of sameness and difference in some kind of tension* (pp.136-137). Similarly, Garber finds in bisexuality *the possibility of* [a] *kind of reading ... that is cumulative and even episodic rather than continuous and given* (p.513). Bisexuality becomes a kind of resistance to closure, or at least to closure as the key to meaning.

Narrating bisexuality thus involves neither, on the one hand, just describing a static moment outside its history, a specular performance, nor, on the other hand, simply a teleological structuring of narrative, in which the ending determines the significance of particular moments that have come before. Bisexual life stories bear the burden of resisting the imperatives of dominant modes of storytelling, resisting notions of fence-sitting, immaturity, and unreliability that are engendered by the focus on monosexual closure, final partnership. Narrating bisexual lives differently, in ways that make meaningful and satisfying sense of bisexual experiences, involves, instead, telling the tensions of an ongoing construction.

While lesbian or classical narratives may resist such a pattern or at least do nothing to foster it, bisexual narratives may invite it. Amending the lesbian coming-out narrative by adding another chapter, the bisexual story destabilises the teleological closure of linear narrative. Many of the women's narratives published in collections like *Closer to Home* and *Plural Desires* describe moving from identifying as lesbian to identifying as bisexual, and Paula Rust's research (1993) confirms that bisexual women are more likely than not to have identified as lesbian in the past (p.44). By conceptualising sexual identity formation as a 'linear, goal-oriented, developmental process', Rust notes, social science research has been unable to account for bisexuality, which was:

> *... either considered nonexistent or conceptualized as an intermediate state between heterosexuality and homosexuality. Bisexual identity, therefore, might be adopted as a stepping stone on the way to homosexual identity ... but was not considered an end in itself.* (p.51)

By undermining the monosexual identity that might have seemed to be the end of the story, however, bisexuality undermines the familiar notion of identities as endings.

Tracing the narratives of bisexuality, especially serial bisexuality, makes evident an imposition of continuous identity that is implied but unnoticed in mono (that is, homo- or hetero-) sexualities. Although bisexuality provides an excellent example of the constraints of identity as conventionally understood, however, it is not the only locus of attempts to narrativise and problematise identity. Another reworking of identity can be found in Minnie Bruce Pratt's *Identity: Skin, Blood, Heart* (1984). Pratt's autobiographical essay traces her understandings of herself as white, woman, Christian-raised, married, southerner, lesbian, poet, and relentlessly emphasises the process of change as she learns about the meanings of these identities, and as she acts upon her knowledge. Biddy Martin and Chandra Mohanty (1986) in their reading of Pratt focus on her moving:

> *...away from the purely personal, visceral experience of identity suggested by the title to a complicated working out of the relationship between home, identity, and community that calls into question the notion of a coherent, historically continuous, stable identity and works to expose the political stakes concealed in such equations.* (p.195)

Pratt discusses how she has:

> *... worked at stripping away layer after layer of my false identity, notions of skin, blood, heart based in racism and anti-Semitism* (p.43),

and notes that

> *.... the process of change is long, and since the unjust world is reduplicated every day, in large and small, so I must try to recreate, every day, a new self striving for a new just world* (p.46).

Pratt's reworking of identity takes her identities, her positions in webs of social and historical relations, as starting points. 'Lesbian', for Pratt, is not the conclusion of a conversion narrative but the beginning of a jump *from my edge and outside myself, into radical change, for love* (p.19). Bisexuality has become a focus for changing understandings of sexuality and identity. Paradoxically, it has done so in part by putting into play the possibility of self-description in terms of a new category. Bisexual identity might seem to suture over these complexities of identity, to posit and emphasise an essence, a self, subject, individual. But it can treat that self-naming not as a conclusion but as an occasion for generating stories, narratives, new ways of reading: the beginning of a jump into radical change.

**Acknowledgements**

Thanks to Ruth Gibian, Adam Dowis, and Alix Schwartz for helpful feedback on drafts of this essay.

# 24

# Bisexuality:

## Some thoughts about privilege

by

Mark Trudinger

Collectively, it seems to me, bisexual people have been a bit unsure about how to discuss privilege – more specifically, how to acknowledge the privileges we do have. We seem to have been more keen to loudly protest the discrimination we face, that double-invisibility we call biphobia. This protest has been for good reason. We face biphobia from gay men and lesbian women, as well as straight people. While part of a culture of heterosexual dominance, biphobia is also part of what's been labelled 'monosexual dominance'. Biphobia is similar, but in some ways more subtle and complex than homophobia, which we also have to deal with (Ochs 1996).

While bisexual people have written and spoken about our experiences of marginalisation and offered fairly detailed examples and analyses of biphobia, we also walk with a certain amount of privilege. What might happen if we found ways of naming that privilege? What further understandings about sexuality politics could we offer? What effects might acknowledging our privileges have on our connections – personally and politically – with gay men and lesbian women, and with straight people?

## A both/and approach to privilege

In protesting our specific location in homo- and biphobia, we've come up with witty, and sometimes grave metaphors, such as: 'If we're queer-bashed, not just half of us hurts'; 'If we're shot outside a queer pub, we don't only half die'; and 'If we're fired, we don't just lose half our jobs'. While these aspects of the injustices that bisexual people face are important to name – and, like broader issues of homophobia, *keep* naming – I wonder if we can also begin to talk more about the privileges we *do* have.

As soon as I write this I start to hesitate: 'Well, maybe, but not at the cost of naming biphobia and the marginalisation we also face'. Perhaps we can find a 'typically bi' solution to the dilemma – to not regard privilege and marginalisation as mutually exclusive, as if we have to acknowledge only one or the other, but to see the issues from the 'both/and' orientation that bisexual people have so strongly articulated in other contexts. Can we both acknowledge the structural and personal discrimination we face and acknowledge the times we walk with privilege? Both are sides of the same coin. As Rebecca Shuster writes:

> *As bisexuals, we hold a position similar to that of the middle class, making it appear as if someone can 'make it' in a system where no-one truly can. We are victimized by the overall system of lesbian/gay oppression and are forced into the role of preserving that system by representing a freedom of choice that cannot fully exist as long as the oppression exists. Therefore, it is vital that we take responsibility as bisexuals for the ways we benefit from the privileges of heterosexuality and simultaneously demand that no-one, including bisexuals, is targeted for being non-heterosexual.* (1992, p.153)

**Privilege as context-specific**

One of the important factors in understanding bisexual people and privilege is that the privileges we walk with are very context-specific. While straight people's heterosexual dominance is context-specific and interwoven with the politics and personal locations of gender, class, and so on, the privileges we as bisexual people enjoy are more personally context-specific depending on our sexual histories, our current partners, and other factors.

For example, I'm currently in a long-term monogamous relationship with a woman. In our circles of friends, on the street, and to my family, I'm usually read as heterosexual. While I rail against this reading, and I sometimes come home alternately angry and despondent on the days when I've felt I've had to 'act straight', or when my sexual identity has been talked about insultingly, it's still the case that my current situation brings with it more privilege than if I were in a relationship with another man, went to queer events more often, or were more 'out' to different people in my life.

Of course, my situation may change, as may many other bisexual folks. So the sexual privileges we enjoy not only differ from person to person, but across time. This doesn't mean, though, that acknowledging and working to dismantle heterosexual privilege is something we should be able to choose to take on or not, as Kathleen Bennett writes:

> *While working with gays and lesbians to fight heterosexism, we must acknowledge the truth that they are far less likely to find themselves in a societally-approved relationship than we are. Our own potential to find such approval, in addition, depends completely on the chance occurrence of whom we happen to fall in love with. The ethical response to this is to live our commitment to fighting heterosexual privilege even, indeed especially, when we are in ostensibly heterosexual relationships. We cannot take safe haven in the 'acceptable' portion of our experience, for our bisexual identity as a whole is socially unacceptable.* (1992, p.227)

In a context that acknowledges the context-specific nature of heterosexual privilege, any discussion of bisexual privilege will largely have to be grounded in one's own personal experience, as I hope to do in the reflections that follow. It may be more useful to talk about heterosexual privilege in the various contexts that we find ourselves in at different points in time, rather than something we simply 'have'. I'm hopeful, however, that, despite our different partners, lifestyles, and so on, bisexual people can somehow find a common language with which to name and talk about sexual privilege.

**Naming the privileges we do have**

Can bisexual people name the privileges we do have, while not silencing the injustices we face and also remembering their context-specificity? I hope that we can. Perhaps a starting place is the privilege of choice. As many people of marginalised groups have pointed out to members of dominant groups, to have a choice in situations often comes from privilege. While biphobia and homophobia impact on the sexual choices of bisexual people, to even have such a choice is a privilege that lesbians and gay men don't have.[1] If we find ourselves in relationships with people of the 'opposite' sex, we can mention their names without fear of rejection or reprisal, as we 'pass' as straight. While much has been written about the sadness, anger, and confusion that 'passing' can bring, it also brings with it certain amounts of safety and other benefits. If we're in relationships with people of the 'opposite' sex, we can get married, have and/or adopt children more easily, and enjoy a range of benefits offered by governments, institutions, people we pass on the street, and our families, that may not be open to lesbians and gay men. I'm aware that issues of choice may sit differently for bisexual people in same-sex relationships. What aspects of privilege might we still be able to name when we find ourselves in same-sex relationships? What other aspects of privilege might we be able to name?

**Honouring the work of lesbians and gay men**

Another set of privileges that could be named are the benefits we enjoy from all the work that gay men and lesbian women have done – and still do, every day. they have created a language with which we can more articulately talk about our identity, about oppression, about sex. They have created a public space for us through marches, rallies, and other activist work; set up services such as safer sex and AIDS clinics; and created queer places to socialise, be relatively free from homophobic harassment, and to party. Yes, bisexual people have been involved in many of these activities from the beginning, often having to hide their bisexuality because of biphobia. But this doesn't take away from the work that thousands of gay men and lesbian women have done to create radical changes that have benefited us as bisexual people.

It feels to me that many times gay men and lesbian women have created changes that we bisexual folk have almost breezed on in and accepted. Sometimes we've also then moved a little too quickly to raising issues of biphobia. I'm reminded here of a workshop a few years ago about 'gay men and straight men talking', where I publicly identified as bisexual and raised issues of biphobia. While taking this stand was important, I'm sure I could have spent more time honouring the work that the gay facilitator had done to create a space for sexuality to be even talked about in the first place.

At other times, gay men and lesbian women have specifically invited us as bisexual people to be part of projects and services, and our issues have been specifically addressed. How often have bisexual groups invited gay men or lesbian women to talk about issues of bisexual privilege? How often have we sought to work in ways that are accountable to gay men and lesbian women so that we don't inadvertently reproduce homophobia or heterosexual dominance? How often have we asked gay men and lesbian women to review the books we have produced? (And, if so, would some of the early bisexual grandstanding – 'I've got the best sexuality because I can have whatever I want' – have gone unchallenged?) Lesbians and gay men also often have helpful ideas about how to raise issues with straight folk, and we could benefit from listening to their experiences.

### Using privilege

> *Some of us live in both the straight and lesbian worlds. Bisexual women can be catalysts for change among heterosexuals ... We can harness resources from heterosexual society and use them toward productive ends. As Audre Lourde has written, privilege (even heterosexual privilege) is not inherently wrong as long as we don't waste it.* (McKeon 1992, p.33)

One of the more apparent times that bisexual folk in relationships with people of the 'opposite' sex can challenge others' assumptions about our sexuality – or can challenge homophobia that might be said in our presence – is when people assume we're straight. As Rebecca Kaplan writes:

> *Compulsory heterosexuality influences the ways in which we are diminished and the ways in which we are treated better when we are seen with men. Both the insults and the so-called compliments must be challenged. We and the men we are with can confront people on their heterocentric assumptions when we encounter them. By doing so, we shake up those assumptions, since people do not expect to have their homophobia confronted by apparent heterosexuals.* (1992, p.277)

Here I'm tempted to make a list of queer-punk/homocore suggestions for direct action – the specific queer subculture and types of activism that I've mostly been involved in – such as unexpected kiss-ins in straight venues but, of course, such a list won't fit for everyone. This reminds me that if our privilege is context-specific in each of our lives, then how we each use our privilege also needs to be in contexts that are specific to each of us.

In the contexts in which we find ourselves in a position of relative privilege, then, how can we *use* these privileges to challenge heterosexual dominance – not necessarily as part of some formal group or movement, but in our everyday lives? How can we use these privileges at work? In our families? What conversations might we need to have with our friends and partners who identify as straight?

## Naming privilege – personal and political consequences

What might be some of the consequences of naming privilege? I would hope that to do so would bring bisexual people closer to gay men and lesbian women – both personally closer and create a space where we can stand more strongly together politically. To break our relative silence on the privileges we do have, to name these in front of gay men and lesbian women, could go some ways to repair past injustices of *not* naming that privilege, and of the times when we have been happy to benefit from the work that gay men and lesbian women have done, without giving something back.

Perhaps naming privilege will also bring us closer to straight people as well. I know that some straight friends interested in issues of power would find it easier to stand with me on issues of sexuality if they heard me talk more often about the privileges I enjoy. There are aspects of straight life, identity, and privilege that we can related to, that we can have compassion for, or that we ourselves also directly experience. Rather than constantly defining ourselves almost as if in opposition to straight people, what spaces might be created if we more regularly 'stood with' straight people, not just in private conversations, but publicly as well?

**Taking other steps**

In my life I've found that taking responsibility for issues of privilege and power has led me to look at other areas of privilege I have. Naming the privileges I do have, and working to understand these, has also been informed by my experiences of marginalisation.

> *Many women, people with disabilities, people who are poor or working class, Jews, lesbians, gays and bisexuals are already competent in two or more cultures. They understand mainstream American culture and are fluent in their own. Sometimes this understanding gives them the impetus to challenge the cultural assumptions of whiteness.*
>
> *It can give them an insight into how the dominance of one culture oppresses and exploits people outside the mainstream.* (Kivel 1996, p.208)

Bisexual groups (in the US at least) have been keen to address issues of racism. Addressing racism, classism, sexism, and so on; these are ongoing issues we can take on as individuals and groups. Where might an approach to taking on issues of sexual privilege lead us as bisexual people, individually and collectively? What other issues do we need to address in our own lives and our communities? What other ripples might we create?

## Acknowledgements

Thanks to the following people who have informed the ideas in this paper, especially *Darlene Corry, David Denborough, Robin Ochs, Maria Pallotta-Chiarolli, Jacinta Toomey*, and *Cheryl White*.

### Note

1. While I've known both lesbians who've had sexual relationships with men, and gay men who've had relationships with women, for ease of writing and reading I use 'lesbian' and 'gay' here in their usual exclusive sense, while fully recognising that this in itself may cover-up some of the complexities and delightful oddities of gender, identity, and sexuality.

# PART SEVEN

# *Transgender / bi-gender experience*

Featuring writings from the Norweigan doctor and family therapist Esben Esther Pirelli Benestad, and young Mexican psychologist Mercedes Martinez, this section attempts to convey some of the complexities posed and possibilities opened by transgender / bi-gender experience.

# 27

# Gender belonging

## Children, adolescents, adults and the role of the therapist

by

Exben Esther Pirelli Benestad

*A heartfelt sigh.*
*For some children the world must be as confusing*
*as a foreign country with the strangest words and habits.*
*However hard they try to live up to these incomprehensible*
*'laws of nature', they cannot succeed.*
(Esther Pirelli, 1999)

## Introduction

In order to materialise inner convictions of gender(s), many grown individuals leave their family, friends, school, and jobs to establish themselves within a context that will affirm their self-experienced gender. This process of 'giving up what one has, to become what one is', has tremendous costs. It is, however, many people's only option for a reasonably good life. The younger the individual, the less potency she/he possesses in order to break away from non-confirming life conditions. Generally, children and adolescents are dependent upon their significant others to stay alive. This poses very particular problems when a child and/or adolescent displays gender in ways that give rise to worry in family members and friends.

Being a public bi-gendered person in the Norwegian landscape of doctors, family therapists and sexologists, I have received testimonies from parents and professionals on the phenomenon that quite a number of children at some point display 'cross gendered' behaviour. Most often, I believe, this is regarded as children's play and experimentation with adult expressions, and thus not conceived as problematic. The more lasting and the more extensive the cross-gendered behaviour becomes, however, the more liable are parents and/or other significant others to worry about the child's future mental health status and the child's future in general.

The extent of cross-gendered behaviour, and people's concerns about it, has given rise to diagnostic evaluations. The DSM IV condition of Gender Identity Disorder in childhood is manifested by four (or more) of the following:

- Repeatedly stated desire to be, or insistence that he or she is, the other sex.
- In boys, preference for cross-dressing or simulating female attire; in girls, insistence on wearing only stereotypical masculine clothing.
- Strong and persistent preferences for cross-sex roles in make-believe play or persistent fantasies of being the other sex.
- Intense desire to participate in the stereotypical games and pastimes of the other sex.
- Strong preference for playmates of the other sex.

In a course description, the DSM-IV states that by late adolescence or adulthood, about three quarters of boys who had a childhood history of 'Gender Identity Disorder' (GID) report a homosexual or bisexual orientation, but without concurrent GID. Most of the remainder report a heterosexual orientation, also without concurrent GID. Some adolescents may develop a clearer cross-gender identification and request sex-reassignment surgery or may continue in a 'chronic course of gender confusion or dysphoria'. For the benefit of the reader, it may be added that the percentages for girls are unknown, due to the scarcity of 'clinical material' on girls with GID in childhood.

Troubled adults will sometimes contact health professionals for advice and/or therapy concerning the cross-gendered behaviour of children. Such contacts are far more frequent if the child is of the somatic male sex. Presently there is no consensus as to how professionals should respond. The Harry Benjamin International Gender Dysphoria Association has, however, produced some general guidelines. The following is from the very recent sixth version (2001) of their Standards of Care concerning the assessment and Treatment of Children and Adolescents with Gender Identity Disorders (GID):

**Phenomenology**

- Gender identity disorders in children and adolescents are different from those seen in adults, in that a rapid and dramatic developmental process (physical, psychological and sexual) is involved. Gender identity disorders in children and adolescents are complex conditions. The young person may experience his or her phenotype sex as inconsistent with his or her own sense of gender identity. Intense distress is often experienced, particularly in adolescence, and there are frequently associated emotional and behavioural difficulties. There is greater fluidity and variability in outcomes, especially in pre-pubertal children. Only a few gender variant youths become transsexual, although many eventually develop a homosexual orientation.

- Commonly seen features of gender identity conflicts in children and adolescents include a stated desire to be the other sex; cross-dressing; play with games and toys usually associated with the gender with which the child identifies; avoidance of the clothing, demeanor and play normally associated with the child's sex and gender of assignment; preference for playmates or friends of the sex and gender with which the child identifies; and dislike of bodily sex characteristics and functions. Gender identity disorders are more often diagnosed in boys.

- Phenomenologically, there is a qualitative difference between the way children and adolescents present their sex and gender predicaments, and the presentation of delusions or other psychotic symptoms. Delusional beliefs about their body or gender can occur in psychotic conditions but they can be distinguished from the phenomenon of a gender identity disorder. Gender identity disorders in childhood are not equivalent to those in adulthood and the former do not inevitably lead to the latter. The younger the child the less certain and perhaps more malleable the outcome.

In these ways, the DSM-IV and Harry Benjamin International Gender Dysphoria Association focus on the child as having a 'mental disorder' for which more effective treatments will be sought in the child's future. And yet, the diagnosis of GID only persists into adolescence or adulthood for approximately one percent of the child population with GID. On the historical evolution of the Harry Benjamin standards of care, it is interesting to observe that the sixth version opens for much more extensive medical treatments at a far younger stage than was the case in version five.

**Challenges and dilemmas**

The diagnostic criteria of the DSM-IV, and the guidelines of the Harry Benjamin International Gender Dysphoria Association, raise many questions. I have listed here a range of challenges and dilemmas that the rest of this article will seek to explore.

- When we know that many children and adults are sufficiently bodily different from the two sex/gender majorities to be excluded from both of them, and a substantial number of grown individuals say that they belong to both or neither, can we meaningfully apply the term 'the other sex'?

- Do present westerns norms relating to perceptions and expressions of gender offer sufficient capacity for people to meet and mirror all mosaics of gender and gender associated human qualities? If not, are we in consequence diagnosing, treating and thus pathologising individuals on the basis of normative shortcomings?

- Do unusual expressions and experiences of gender and/or sexual orientation predispose suffering on their own account, or are the problems experienced by those in question due to lack of affirmation?
- When is it right to question the reality of subjective experiences?
- Shall we use terms like 'gender disturbed' in the first place, or should we rather say that some expressions of gender disturb?
- If some human beings are equipped with combinations of qualities that cannot as of yet be contained and positively reflected within interacting human cultures, what ethics shall guide clinicians?
- Is it ethical to address the unusually equipped child for change, or must the therapeutic challenge be to address the shortcomings within the common perceptions of gender?
- Is it possible to construct recommendable modes of action for professionals and societies to prevent misfortunes like suicide, self-mutilation, self-disqualifications, self-denial, alcohol and drug abuse, psychiatric and social problems for those who may fail to achieve a sense of belonging for their special gender(s) and/or sexual orientation(s)?

I will return to these questions and dilemmas at a later stage in this paper.

**The fate of children with cross-gendered behaviour**

The number of children displaying significant cross-gendered behaviour is between 3-4% of the child population. Only a very small number of those diagnosed with GID in childhood grow into adult trans-people. More are likely to become gay, lesbian or bisexual.

Research has shown that a large percentage (70-80%) of homosexual men and lesbian women have displayed cross-gendered behaviour to a degree that could qualify as GID in childhood (Carrier 1986). In this way, homosexual men and lesbian women can, to a large degree, be recognised in childhood on the grounds of cross-gendered behaviour. This group of young people approaches a perilous adolescence. Research has proved that lesbian and homosexual (and trans) adolescents face a tough time, including a much higher risk of suicide than same aged heterosexuals (Hegna, Kristiansen & Moseng, 1999).

It is possible to recognise in childhood a group of people who are likely to undergo difficult times in their adolescence. It is therefore also possible to take some action regarding this. It is my belief that we have a responsibility to try to prevent the hardships that we know will face many young gay and lesbian and trans-people. In order to prevent these hardships we must first endeavour to understand the complexities of gender identity.

**Understanding gender – definitions of words and concepts**

The use of words and concepts about gender are diverse. There are multitudes of words and multitudes of meanings that these words convey. In the professional world and in the lay world, there is often confusion about words and concepts. People may be using the same words but their connotations may be divergent. Consider, for instance, the word 'feminine'. This is a word that denotes meanings ranging from the behaviour of some women, to the behaviour of some gay men, to the shape of human bodies. Is the term 'womanly' the same as 'feminine'? Is 'manly' the same as 'masculine'? Is a 'female body' the same as a 'feminine' one, and can a body be both 'female' and 'masculine'?

Our perceptions of our gender are based upon our own experiences and the conceptual offerings or tools we glean from our surroundings. When recognisable offerings of words and concepts are unavailable, the individual must develop her, his or her/his own constructs, or else she/he will suffer feelings of not being 'Right' or, at worst, not being at all.

A route to self-understanding that requires new constructions of words and concepts is hardly to be expected from children and/or adolescents. Children are dependent upon tools offered by the adult world. One professional task therefore is to develop new, and to re-cultivate old words and concepts, to describe all different present and emerging phenomena in 'Genderland' in a recognisable way for all those involved.

Because of the importance of clarity in relation to words and concepts, I feel it is important to offer here a range of descriptions and definitions. These words and concepts serve as a back-drop to ways of understanding gender.

- **Somatic sex** refers to the body as it appears from the outside. The somatic body of the newborn child may be female, male, hermaphroditic or of configurations not congruent with any of the three. Somatic sex generally defines, through the observations of others, the individual's social gender status. It is a powerful level of gender confirmation, however it is based upon external perceptions (Almaas & Benestad 1993).

- **Reproductive sex** refers to the individual's procreative capacity, be it utilised or not utilised. The four variations are as follows. Able or formerly able to become a mother, able or formerly able to become a father, able or formerly able to become both mother and father (theoretically possible for some hermaphrodites) and at no time able to become either mother or father. Reproductive sex cannot be changed. It serves for some as a most important gender affirmation (particularly for those with body/identity congruence), but can sometimes bring painful experiences for those with transgendered qualities and for those without reproductive sex (Almaas & Benestad 2001).

- **Gender identity** refers to a person's basic sense of self as woman or man, or both as woman and man, or neither. The formation of gender identity is profoundly influenced by the common frames of woman/man. Gender identity is generally stable after the pre-school years but for some it may change over time (Almaas & Benestad 1993). Gender identity is a very powerful level of gender confirmation, as it may overthrow both somatic sex and body consciousness (Almaas & Benestad1993; Zucker et al. 1999).

- **Body consciousness** refers to an individual's sense of contact with her, his, her/his or a different kind of body. The gendered body consciousness includes contact and experience with one's own genitals and other gendered body parts. Body consciousness can be impaired when for instance the individual has been the victim of sexual offence, or when there is incongruence between the experienced gender and the experienced body. The body consciousness can be that of female, male, hermaphroditic or that of a different kind of body, and it is a powerful level of gender confirmation (Almaas & Benestad 1993).

➢ **Body picture** refers to what we ordinarily display in public. If the somatic body could be seen as a box that can contain any gender, the body picture is that box in wrappings. The body picture can on the somatic side, be of female, male, intermediate (hermaphroditic) shape, or in the shape of a non-gendered kind of body. On the cultural side, the 'wrappings' may signal feminine, masculine, androgynous or non-gendered qualities. Body picture is the level of gender confirmation that is most easily manipulated as for instance in cross-dressing. Body picture is a means by which we can relate to the world around us and seek affirmation (Almaas & Benestad 1993).

➢ **Gender role** refers to the range of interests, choices, manners, actions, styles that are generally perceived and defined by society as masculine or feminine. By referring to gender roles in this way however, it implies that gender roles are completely arbitrary, a view that would not be universally shared by all researchers in the field (Sullivan, Bradley & Zucker 1995). It is widely accepted however that the same individual may perform both feminine and masculine traits, and thus be androgynous in terms of role. Prior to the influence of feminism and gay liberation movements, gender role within western countries had powerful gender confirming properties, but as the norms of gender roles have widened and multiplied, their power of gender confirmation has lessened. However, some somatic females experiencing both female and male gender identity, seek gender confirmation through what are considered masculine actions like mountain climbing, and soccer playing. Some somatic male transvestites/cross-dressers/trans-people refuse to engage in masculine activities when dressed.

➢ **Sexual orientation** refers to a person's orientational mode of responsiveness to gendered stimuli. An individual may be turned on by and/or fall in love with only (if not all) females, with only (if not all) males, with both (if not all) females and males and/or with hermaphrodites, cross-dressers, transgendered or other individuals with no specific belonging within the existing norms of gender.

Some people are indifferent to gendered stimuli and can be seen as asexual. Gender orientation is otherwise labelled heterosexual, homosexual, lesbian or bisexual. The labelling is generally based upon descriptions by others, and may change when viewed from the individual's own perspective. A transsexual with male somatic body may consider herself heterosexual, while from an outside view, 'he is homosexual'. Sexual orientation plays important roles in gender confirmation/affirmation. Sexual orientation is not necessarily stable over time (Almaas & Benestad 1993; Sullivan, Bradley & Zucker 1995).

- **Gender belonging** refers to the permanent or temporary state of confirmed, or at best affirmed, gender. Gender confirmation/affirmation operates on seven levels: somatic body, reproductive sex, gender identity, body consciousness, body picture, gender role and sexual orientation. The options of gender belonging are as female, male, male and female, transgendered or other (not as of yet denoted). Gender belonging is the goal of gender confirming experiences and behaviours, and it may change over time. A positive gender belonging is to be perceived and approved of by others the same way as one perceives and approves of one self as gender. Most trans-people go through a process seeking a positive gender belonging that is congruent with their self-experienced gender identity (Almaas & Benestad 1993; Doorn 1997).

- **Gender cruising** refers to an increasing tendency for individuals to blend, to try out, to renew, to cultivate and experiment with gendered expressions. Gender cruising includes females functioning in 'typical male' settings, and males in typical 'female' ones, but also individuals who in many ways are transcending gender as we thus far have perceived it. Gender cruising may be deliberately in opposition to the culturally imposed dichotomy of gender, and/or an intended or unintended means of gender confirmation (Almaas & Benestad 1999).

- **Gender crossing** refers to the crossing from one gender, either permanently or in a back and forth mode, to another. Gender crossing ordinarily abides by the norms of dualistic gender conceptions (Almaas & Benestad 1993).

- **Biological gender** refers to biological substrates for different concepts of gender. The Darwinistic perspective uses biological gender in reference to the ability of procreation. Some workers in the field of transgender link biological gender to gender identity in so far that it influences aspects of the central nervous system, while others link biological gender to the presence or absence of specific gendered bodily qualities. The term is one which is accompanied by discussion in relation to what in the diverse world of gender is actually determined or influenced by that which is referred to as biology (Almaas & Benestad 1999).

➢ **Gender dichotomy** refers to the concept that only two distinct sexes and/or genders exist, with no other scientifically or culturally accepted alternatives. The dichotomy is strongly and subversively supported by sentences and expressions like: 'the opposite sex', 'the opposite gender', 'gender crossing', 'cross-dressing', and so on. In gender related scientific literature, the dichotomy appears in sentences and conceptions like: 'to label oneself boy or girl', 'man or woman', 'to be confused or uncertain whether one is boy or girl', 'the basic sense of self as either a male or female', and many, many others.

➢ **Body dysphoria** describes the subjective experience of having a body that does not confirm inner conceptions of, for example, gender. Body dysphoria is widespread in that an ever increasing number of people are discontent with their bodies and/or their body parts, giving multiple challenges to cosmetic industries and/or plastic surgeons (Almaas & Benestad 1999). Body dysphoria can also take the form of 'discomfort with sexual anatomy', 'aversion of anatomical features' (Blanchard & Steiner 1990), and 'long standing feeling of being uncomfortable with their anatomically designated sex' (Sullivan, Bradley & Zucker 1995).

➢ **Intersex conditions and ambiguous genitalia.** In the medical culture, children who are born with somatic intersex and/or ambiguous genitalia are considered misshapen or deformed, even though intersexed adult individuals claim their right to be – as they are. These people represent 'third alternatives' on the somatic body scale and they comprise a substantial number of people who cannot and will not abide to the dichotomised standards of somatic gender.

➢ **Sex and gender paradigms**. Supported by science, law, religion and common beliefs, there exist paradigms as to what are the 'right' combinations of sex, gender, love behaviour, sexual behaviour, sexual and gendered expressions. These paradigms are being deconstructed under, amongst many, the scrutinising eyes of the transgendered and intersexed societies.

➢ **Genderland** refers to the well established and utilised means of communication, and growing self-consciousness, within the totality of different 'transgendered societies'. The multitude of internet links concerning issues on cross-dressing, sex and gender beautifully illustrate this multinational society.

**Responding to children and adolescents with unusual gender expressions**

Having considered these terms and the complexities of issues of gender, now let us return to the question of how to respond to children and adolescents with unusual gender expressions.

Gender cruising, cross-gendered or transgendered behaviours and expressions by children, adolescents and young adults often disturb the significant others in their lives. In some situations this occurs to the point that some parents, family members and other adults seek professional help in order to treat and/or to help these unusual individuals with their possible problems of gender identities and/or sexual orientations.

This raises a number of ethical questions. Is there ethical validity in treating GID children when their behaviour is non-conforming and yet benevolent? Is there ethical validity in treating an early sign of homosexuality, a human condition which is as sound as heterosexuality? What's more, although, in a majority of cases, cross-gendered expressions in childhood foregoes homosexual identification in later life (Green 1968, 1974, 1987; Sullivan, Bradley & Zucker 1995; Zucker et al. 1999), quite often children who display significant cross-gendered expressions develop into adults who experience themselves as ordinarily gendered heterosexuals. It is therefore very difficult to prove 'therapeutic' effects from individual child therapy on individual's future gender behaviour and on their self-concepts of gender.

Nevertheless, therapy is being offered to these individuals and rarely is the validity of these individually focused therapeutic interventions questioned

(Sullivan, Bradley & Zucker 1995; Zucker et al. 1999). There has been little comparison or elaboration of the type of interventions offered due to the limited number of researchers who have addressed the problems of the young (Bradley & Zucker 1997). What is clear is that no therapeutic measure has proved significantly influential in relation to the quality of life for the individuals in question. Nor has anyone been able to prove effects from the therapeutic intervention on the individual adult 'choices' of gender identity and/or sexual orientation.

Attempts to impose gender identity upon individuals have proven difficult if not impossible. In the John/Joan case, a somatic boy had his penis destroyed by accident before he was a year old. Under medical assistance and therapeutic supervision, the family brought the child up as a girl. Nevertheless he never accepted to be a she, and returned to male status in his teens (Diamond & Sigmundson 1997). There is a lack of scientific proof as to any possible benefits of influencing gender identity and/or sexual orientation. This is due partly to the inapplicability of positivistic scientific methods to a field with such a small number of clients and when a long duration of time is required for observation. In addition, approaching gender identity and belonging as if gender is a quality which is in some way individually inherent, may in the future be seen to be problematic. Applying therapeutic measures on unusual combinations of somatic bodies and gender identities may also come to be seen as unethical.

Given these grave uncertainties concerning the appropriateness of individual therapy with children or adolescents who display transgendered behaviours and experiences; and given the knowledge that many of the same young people will experience painful disapproval from the world around them; I have become convinced of the importance of focusing on the networks of these children and young people rather than upon individuals themselves.

**Requests for help**

As a public bi-gendered doctor, I have the privilege of being contacted by people from different parts of Norway concerning children and adolescents with transgendered expressions and behaviours. These young people are referred by adults of their family-network and/or by various health professionals. My task has developed into finding some mode of action that could render these children/adolescents some positive support on their life paths. In the process, I have had to ask myself a number of basic questions. Firstly, 'Who is in trouble? Those who refer these individuals, or the individuals themselves?' The answer to this question is naturally both, since the trouble of the first, will necessarily affect the latter. A second basic question has been: 'Are these individuals best helped by coming to me, or can I accomplish more by addressing them where they live?' And a third basic question has been: 'Do I address the children/adolescents directly, do I address them through their network, or do I create both-and solutions?'

## A therapeutic 'policy' – treating the world

Based on the understandings articulated earlier in this paper, and confirmed by the fact that it was not the individuals themselves, but troubled adults who sought help, I have formulated the following the therapeutic 'policy':

The individual who displays transgendered behaviour does not suffer from any disease and shall thus not be treated. Her/his main source of pain and trouble is the way she/he is met and perceived by the world. One main consequence of this malignant interaction is the transgendered person's feeling of self-contempt and the absence of gender belonging. The main therapeutic route to a better situation for the 'identified' transgendered individual is thus to treat her/his world of significant others. For the non-identified transgendered person, for instance children who display cross-gendered behaviour, the therapeutic route is to prepare their surroundings for what may be likely to occur in the development of the individual. The main route to a better life for many unidentified transgendered people is therefore to 'treat the world'. A major proportion of young people with transgendered expressions will grow into homosexuals or lesbians and need no therapy on those grounds. They are, however, in urgent need of support in an often quite hostile world.

In situations where is it clear that the individuals themselves are seeking assistance, this assistance is generally not needed to relieve them of a 'gender problem', but to try to facilitate some meaningful sense of gender belonging, and to reduce and at best dissolve their experience of body dysphoria. My contact with young self identified transgendered individuals has taught me that we cannot place upon them the burden of comprehending an uncomprehending world of significant adults. As one individual said to me: 'I really hate it when someone asks me to understand everybody else's problem with me, I have quite enough trying to understand myself'.

Thus the challenge for all health professionals, and indeed for all adults, could be formulated as follows: The quest is not for the possibly transgendered child or adolescent to understand or take care of the world, but for the world to understand and take care of the transgendered. More directly, the challenge for us as health professionals seems to be to try to ensure that individuals displaying unusual expressions of gender have a chance to experience a sense of positive gender belonging. To do so, we must work with the networks of significant others.

**Belonging**

The search for a feeling of belonging is basic to the human state, and must be considered very seriously when addressing expressions of gender. The term belonging is widely used. So much of human behaviour concerns attempts to achieve a sense of belonging in a group, in a society, in a family, in a partnership or in the world. The impetus to belong can be recognisable within common expressions like: 'feeling at home', being 'seen', being 'noticed', being 'loved as one is'. Positive belonging is to be perceived and approved by others in the same way as one perceives and approves oneself. The experience of not belonging is very painful and can give rise to self-denial, self-contempt and in the worst cases to suicidal thoughts and actions.

Many transgendered adults, and many individuals with unusual sexual orientation(s), have experienced an almost total lack of affirmation, and thus a lack of positive belonging. This void is, for many, their main source of pain and suffering. Their struggle with themselves is experienced as a struggle induced by their surroundings and by their bodies – the surroundings by not accepting them the way they experience themselves to be, and their body by rendering them a denial of their internally experienced gender. Many people, including Jan Morris in *Conundrum* (1997) and Tracey O'Keefe in *Trans-ex-u-all*; have described the experience of 'I felt I belonged nowhere' (1997).

Finding ways for children who have unusual gender expressions to have better options of experiencing a positive sense of belonging in their life and future has become the basic goal of my work.

**Networking with possibly transgendered individuals**

In 'treating the world' of the possibly transgendered child, it seems important to recognise our responsibilities in guiding the process of identity formation for children and adolescents. Whatever actions we take involve guiding in some direction, so it seems relevant to think through what we understand to be 'good guiding'. Good guiding, to me, involves appreciating all gender expressions and/or expressions of sexual orientations for their own equal worth, and thus to an optimal degree trying to interact positively with the growing individual on her/his/her-his own premises. As a therapist, the tool available to me in this endeavour is networking, and networking seems best done on the location where the individual in question lives.

The current status of networking with possibly transgendered people in most western countries seems to consist of:

1) In most places there seems to be no professionally educated network. Possibly transgendered people are generally left to media, insufficient encyclopaedias and the internet for information and offers of belonging. This option is, to say the least, insufficient.

2) In some circumstances the network of significant others is passively influenced by professionals through statements such as: 'Return when your child is old enough for possible (medical) treatment'.

3) In some circumstances, networks are actively influenced by professionals in a negative manner through statements such as: 'We shall get this idea out of your child's head'.

When I am approached about a possibly transgendered child, the object of my work is to make it more probable for the growing individual to remain within her/his network – regardless of her/his/hir experience and expression of gender and/or sexual orientation. To achieve this aim, my preferred choice is to professionally network with parents, siblings, friends, and professional significant others (teachers, psychologists, psychiatrists, social workers, state officials) and any other individual or group with whom it would be useful to have contact. Where the individual in question clearly indicates her/his transgenderism, it is wise to involve other reflected transvestites, transgenderists and transsexuals in the network. When the individual self-identifies as transgendered, and is actively seeking contact and/or is more than thirteen years of age, he/she is addressed individually or in company with self-chosen significant other(s). Individual therapy is deliberately not offered to children/adolescents under the age of thirteen, in order not to label or stigmatise individuals who are too young for their lives to be understood through adult standards.

For the last two years I have practised this mode of action in Norway and have offered seminars to which I invite present and future teachers of the particular child, child/adolescent psychologists/psychiatrists, social workers, state officials and/or parents/family members.

**Network seminars**

The children and adolescents who display cross-gendered behaviour whom I am presently professionally involved with include seventeen somatic boys ranging from 6 to 17 years of age and one somatic girl of 15. This group of young people ranges across a wide spectrum of experiences from individuals who are grappling with major psychological and social problems to well-functioning children in loving and supportive families. The graver the existing problems concerning the individuals in question, the greater the need for meetings, network seminars and at times individual work with the child or adolescent in question.

My approach in the network seminars involves first and foremost focusing on the cultural shortcomings concerning conceptions of gender and gender expressions, and what problems these pose for those who experience and/or express their gender in uncommon ways. Children and adolescents with trans-expressions need support to develop strategies to maximise positive interactions in an uncomprehending world. They also need support to care for their own flexibility within the realm of gender and gender expressions. The networks of significant others need tools of understanding in order to comprehend their interactions with unusual children and adolescents. For instance, rejection from significant others, and from society as such, can give rise to resistance. In some situations, children and adolescents may develop what I call 'gender defiance', where there exists no other solution than the one primarily decided. For these young people rejection can turn life into a fierce fight to become their self-experienced gender. The resulting rigidity can be of great harm if the individual enters eventual irreversible (medical) sex/gender confirming processes. Less defiance might have rendered openings for other gendered options and a slower pace in the process.

Networking on behalf of transing children and adolescents seems to reduce the unease and tension that has previously been linked to the unusual gender expressions. I experience improved interactions, less teasing and mocking and an improved gender awareness and assertiveness concerning all involved. Having professionals take part in these seminars has spread an improved understanding of gender.

By reducing the fear of the possible transgendered or homo-erotic future for the individuals in question, and by rendering recognisable the insights and knowledge of those concerned, this networking seems to release good energies and actions in all those involved.

## Answers to questions on basic challenges and dilemmas

At the beginning of this paper I posed a series of basic challenges and dilemmas. Here I will seek to offer some answers to these questions.

- A substantial number of individuals do not conform to the dichotomised either/or conceptions of sex and gender. There is basis for expressions like 'another sex/another gender', but the phrase 'the other sex' seems to have reached its date of expiration.
- A substantial number of individuals, on grounds of bodily and/or

psychological qualities, do not meet the overwhelmingly common conceptions on sex and gender. These individuals face a crisis of gender belonging, because they cannot be positively mirrored in an uncomprehending society.

- The shortcomings of western culture that result in a lack of affirmation for a substantial number of individuals, give rise to diagnoses that in turn stigmatise and pathologise this group of individuals.
- A substantial number of adults with unusual gendered bodies and/or unusual self-perceptions of gender, describe their lives as very satisfying. They do, however, underline that vast amounts of rejection and failing comprehension has played a painful part in their lives.
- This substantial number of adults, who cannot be diagnosed as psychotic, but whose genders are unusual, experience significant others claiming to know more about their gender than they themselves. The concepts of the majority seem to attempt to overthrow the subjective experiences of the minority. However this attempt meets with no success.
- There is a substantial and ever growing body of evidence that supports the understanding that individuals thus far diagnosed as having GID, are not themselves disturbed, but do disturb their world of significant others.
- It seems timely for everybody in general, and for therapists in particular, to expand the norms as to what genders and what expressions of gender should be contained and positively reflected in human societies.
- Concerning the substantial number of children and adolescents who display unusual gender expressions, therapists should address the world of significant others aiming to generate a more expanded understanding of sex and gender in these networks, rather than addressing the unusual individual themselves.
- Presently, it is perilous to be an individual of unusual gender(s) and/or sexual orientation(s). The perils include misfortunes like suicide, self-mutilation, self-disqualifications, self-denial, alcohol and drug abuse, psychiatric and social problems. Until the vast array of gendered expressions can be as appreciated in society as the common expressions of the gender majorities

and heterosexuality, therapists should focus their therapeutic actions not at the individuals in question, but on their world of significant others.

## The broader context: changes in the adult world of gender expressions and/or sexual orientations

Over recent years, in Norway and other western countries, there have been some remarkable changes on the 'gender scene'. Now, not only do we see individuals shifting from heterosexuality into lesbianism or homosexuality, but we also see individuals changing from a lesbian- or a homosexual-understanding of self to a transsexual understanding of self. Some formerly heterosexual individuals, with or without transgendered experiences or expressions in their life history, also develop into cross-dressers and/or transsexuals. The claim that, 'they really were like that all the time', is not necessarily confirmed by the individuals in question. These experiences are giving rise to questions about the 'certainty' and the 'permanence' of heterosexual, lesbian and homosexual belongings. The older and more accepted belongings may have served functions as intermediate 'havens' on a longer path in Genderland. All these experiences utterly question and confuse issues as to how we ought to respond to children or adolescents, and for what purpose, in this human world of genders.

Over the last few decades there has also been a profound change in the options available to understand and 'diagnose' unusual gender expressions and/or sexual orientations. The term homosexuality for instance has been on the move. In the first editions of the DSM, homosexuality itself was a diagnosable condition. In the DSM-III this changed but 'Ego-dystonic homosexuality' remained which was characterised by people being 'distressed about his/her sexual orientation'. In the current DSM-IV homosexuality is no longer a category of pathology (Sullivan, Bradley & Zucker 1995). Over the same time, the category of homosexual has been claimed by individuals and entire communities as a statement of intent, identity and pride.

Homosexuality is no longer a feasible term of pathological diagnosis and yet many claim it as an identity category. The terms 'gender identity disorder' and 'transsexuality' remain as terms of diagnosis, but the medical/psychological tendency to pathologise unusual self-concepts of gender and/or unusual gender expressions is decreasing. Categorisations can be helpful in some circumstances. These categories offer the individual words and concepts for a recognition of self which is basic for the development of gender belonging. Within the medical realm, to have categories available as diagnostic tools is sometimes very significant. For instance, the diagnostic category of transsexuality is necessary as a background for hormonal and surgical gender confirming therapy (also called sexual reassignment surgery [SRS]). Even though transsexuality in and of itself should not qualify as a term of pathology, categories of identity are required in order to enable individuals to undergo processes of revelation and to become who they wish to become. How to facilitate these processes of revelation and to enable categories of identity to be empowering concepts rather than terms of pathology, is one of the challenges of this area. Homosexuals and lesbians lost their disease stigma long ago, primarily through their own efforts, and the transgendered are presently fighting to get rid of theirs.

On the international gender scene, the former concepts of transgenderisms with accompanying needs for hormonal and surgical assistance, are persisting, while in addition, new concepts of gender(s) and new gender expressions are emerging with significant effects. The need for sexual reassignment surgery (SRS) for instance, reportedly declines when other, less dichotomised, options of gender are on offer (Van der Ven 1998). There is an increasing recognition that seeking a sense of gender belonging is a process that for many people lasts for years, decades and sometimes entire life-spans.

Gender crossing still exists, while gender cruising is expanding. One location of gender belonging is not necessarily permanent or very long lasting. And yet, there are ongoing reports of beneficial hormonal and surgical gender confirming procedures down to the age of sixteen, when the individual in question has shown substantial signs of classical transsexualism since childhood (Doorn, Gooren, Cohen-Kettenis, Verschoor & Kuiper 1995). While pathology is being challenged, old concepts of transsexualism have survived while many new concepts are also emerging.

The hermaphrodites, the 'both-ands' and the 'owners' of alternatively sexed/gendered bodies are claiming their right to exist and to be counted within the healthy human flock, without having to be forced into the present western dichotomy of gender. Adrianne Dana, presenter at the Third International

Congress on Sex and Gender (Oxford, England, Sept. 1998) expresses these experiences as follows: 'In the United States, transgenderism, as an expandable category, acts as an umbrella concept, which subsumes and accommodates a spectrum of gender, sexual, and social identities and communities'.

This expanding world of growing sex and gender diversity is the present haven for those of us who have come to experience ourselves as not fitting within the common concepts of gender.

**The future**

Living in societies where there are but two options of gender, many experience themselves at a definite crossroads where they have to choose, both in their inner world and in their many interactions with others, to be either man or woman. This choice is definitely limited, in view of the existing multitude of grown individuals in this world who do not experience either of these two options apt. For those experiencing societally incongruent gender(s), there is a need for positive ambivalence; a chance to sense, to try out, to gender cruise, to wait for more certainty for as long as is individually needed. In this process, where the individual is expressing her/his/hirs transgendered feelings, there is a need to meet other reflected transgendered individuals in addition to all those who are gender conforming.

As mentioned previously, many transgendered people experience body dysphoria. Through permission to express one's own sense of being, to develop freely in one's own process, there seems to be a better chance for the individual to experience good relations with their own body. Whatever the status of that body might be, or might be developed into, there is a need for positive body consciousness. It is very late to wait for profound body alterations, before one can experience and learn about one's own body signals. Since the search for gender belonging is experienced by many as a lifelong process with a multitude of implications, there is always a time to dwell within what is presently accessible.

This paper is based on numerous meetings, interviews and discussions with transgendered and intersexed individuals from countries around the globe. In addition, it is based on clinical experiences with transgendered individuals.

My material is not extensive, but it is qualitatively broad and growing, and it renders perspectives on how to address young and possibly transgendered individuals.

Within the professional world there continues to be a tendency to focus on transgendered individuals as ill and problematic, instead of realising the possible shortcomings of both cultural and therapeutic ways of addressing the diversities of human genders. The gender world contains many insights into the existence of healthy transgendered individuals. These insights are better shared within the boundaries of Genderland than on the outside. The professional world is underdeveloped when it comes to the understanding and acceptance of human gender diversity.

There is a great need for the insights and ideas of transgendered people of all kinds to be shared among those whose profession can add to impairment or alleviation of these individuals' life processes. There is an urgent need to co-ordinate efforts so that professionals working with transgender people understand the complexities of the issues concerned. This is imperative, especially for those transgender people who rely on professional expertise to alter their bodies by surgical routes, to bring their gender into alignment with their gender identity.

I envisage a future in which small groups of informed professionals can move to wherever they are needed, to teach and inform different local groups of professionals and/or significant others how to understand and address children or adolescents with unusual gender experiences and expressions. This endeavour will require a willingness to listen to the subjective experiences from the transgendered world and an openness and willingness from the transgendered themselves to share their insights with networks of others.

# 28

# About the expected expert

by

Mercedes Martinez

When I first saw her name in the diary that records my consultations I couldn't have predicted to what extent working with Catherine was going to stretch my world and influence my incipient steps into therapeutic work. Catherine is a transgendered male to female woman; at the moment she is going through the hormone replacement therapy to prepare herself for the operation that is going to happen sometime next year and which will allow her to fulfil her life-long aspiration. However, the multiple steps that Catherine has taken towards gradually inhabiting the world in accordance to her preferred female identity have not gone without difficulties and hardships.

Many of the things that we talked about in our initial meetings had to do with the public's ignorance, fear, and bias against transgendered people. At different times we discussed some of the effects resulting from people's incomprehension and lack of disposition to understand what this 'condition' (to use Catherine's own expression) is about. The fact that Catherine hasn't been able to find a partner is just one of those effects; one that was really afflicting Catherine the first time we met. Loneliness, depression and rejection were a big part of the picture too. But just as strongly featured Catherine's determination and optimism to follow her sense of who she is and has been, and to take the steps to more fully become who she has always wished to be.

In one of our meetings the issue of the lack of appropriate services was addressed. She pointed out the fact that there is hardly anything that responds to the specific needs of transgender people who are often just put into the same sack with all those whose identities do not conform to the more clearly defined categories of heterosexual, gay, lesbian or bisexual: 'We're not homosexual or bisexual, we're not cross dressers – to me clothes are clothes – we're transgendered and I'm heterosexual ... well, it depends on how you see it. It's very complicated.'

Catherine spoke about how she believed some of the issues and concerns that she has could only be fully understood by another transgendered person, someone who knew about the joys and difficulties of such an experience. In a couple of instances Catherine said that I probably could not understand her experience and on occasions was almost apologetic for having presented to me with such a complex situation.

In our third meeting we talked about the history of how Catherine became aware of her female identity, including what it took for her to get an understanding of her experience, the steps that she took to gradually impersonate that identity, and the reactions of acceptance and rejection that different people presented her with. After all of that, Catherine said that next time she wanted to discuss the issue of breaking the news of her undergoing process of change to her daughter, Mary, who lives in another state and is coming to visit her this Christmas. Mary knows nothing about Catherine's situation. Catherine thought that I could tell her how to go about giving Mary the news and how to handle the reactions that may arise as a result, given that I work as a part of counselling teams. The impression that I got from what Catherine said was that this 'problem' was being offered to me as a concession or some sort of compensation for the difficult situation that she put me through by presenting me [illegible] the complexities of her transgendered experience. This time she was counting on my expertise around dealing with these sort of relationship and family issues.

At the start of our following meeting I checked and Catherine was still interested in addressing the issue about breaking the news to her daughter. She spoke about having had a telephone conversation where she had dropped some hints, but was still too uncertain about how Mary would receive the news.

Catherine was very much concerned about the possibility of ruining Mary's plans for her visit at Christmas. Catherine explained that Mary is entering a very important competition for which she has worked very hard and her fear was that the news would upset her so much that it would affect her performance. She was also really worried about being rejected by Mary. At the same time, Catherine spoke with determination about not being willing to go back on the steps she has already taken or to contemplate the possibility of staying how she is right now, in the middle of the process. So, regardless of anybody's reactions, she could only see herself moving forward in this transformation. 'I'm so far advanced in what I am ... she's going to find out eventually'.

This conversation led us again to the place where it had started: Catherine wanted me to tell her how to break the news to Mary and how to handle the different situations that may arise. My answer was that I could not tell her how to do it, but that maybe we could talk about what she thought was important for her daughter to know. I said that I would then write down her exact words so that they were available for her to go back to when the time came. She accepted hesitantly. My guess at the time was that her hesitance spoke to her unmet expectations of receiving my expert advice on the matter.

The thinking behind my suggestion to go in this direction had to do with the understanding that Catherine had taken a position with regard to her life and her identity that was grounded on a very rich history. I had heard about her hopes for her life and also about her commitments to care and consideration for others. My thought was that perhaps having a document that reminded her of all that she stood for could be useful to have when the time came. I hoped that it might be helpful in preventing those arguments such as not needing to explain herself to her daughter because she is the parent and the adult in that relationship, which seemed to make themselves most available in difficult times.

These sorts of arguments definitely did not represent properly all the values, commitments and the history that were informing Catherine's position or honour the care and consideration expressed in her anticipation and preparation for the event. So I started asking questions that referred to that history and some of Catherine's hopes and I wrote her answers down literally.

As we finished the document, we were also approaching the end of our meeting and the time for my next appointment. I asked Catherine how the conversation had gone for her, if she thought that what we did was at all helpful. She had a look of disappointment on her face and her answer was that she still didn't know how she was going to tell her daughter the news or how she was going to manage her reactions. I felt that I had not offered something that had turned out to be useful for Catherine so decided that I could not possibly leave it like that. Noticing that there was still no sign of the next person whom I was meant to see, I asked Catherine if she wanted to go on until the person arrived and she agreed. Frankly, at this point I was already exhausted and I didn't really have an idea as to where to go from there. My understanding was that Catherine was still expecting to hear from me suggestions about how to handle the situation with her daughter but it was clear that I couldn't respond to that request. I remember that I took a deep breath and it must have been then that my mind found a little clarity.

I asked Catherine if she had already told someone else, maybe a friend or another relative, about what was going on for her. She said that she had told two of her friends. Catherine spoke about how these events had gone and I asked questions about what had actually happened, how she had chosen to proceed, how she had responded to the reactions from those people, what sort of thinking informed those decisions and the intentions and purposes behind her thoughts and actions. It was then possible to use the description of these two previous situations as a reference to compare to what she would do similarly or differently with regard to her daughter.

Three quarters of an hour later when I told Catherine that we should be finishing she said, 'You know what, I've gotten more from this 45 minutes than from all the sessions we've had before'. Due to the time constraint it was not possible to talk a lot more about this so I only asked a few questions, including, if it would be all right to send her a letter that spoke about our meeting. I had already introduced this possibility in previous sessions and she thought that would be a good idea.

This is the letter that I wrote before I saw Catherine again.

*Hello Catherine,*

*Late but sure, the announced letter is here. My intention in writing it is to share some reflections and offer some questions that didn't get the time to be said in our session. So, here it goes.*

*At the very end of our last meeting you said that you had gotten more out of the last 45 minutes than of the previous four sessions. When I asked you what had been different or more helpful you said that the questions had brought forward what you already knew about ways of dealing with situations of 'breaking the news' to other people and also dealing with their reactions. You added something like, 'it's not about this being the right way or the wrong way, it's the way I know'.*

*I was left with lots of ideas in my mind so I'm glad that I can write them down now. First of all, do you reckon it would be helpful to talk a bit more about those things that were brought forward by the questions?*

*I was also left wondering what other knowledges you might have regarding other issues that you've mentioned in our meetings like dealing with rejection or countering the effects of depression. Are there things that make it easier or harder to remember those knowledges that you have?*

*Do you have any ideas of what sort of questions I could be asking that would make it easier to remember or bring forward your knowledges?*

*Well, that's basically it. But just before I finish, I'd like to say that I'm glad we went for another 45 minutes the last time we met. They seemed to be more useful for you and for me they've represented a great opportunity for reflection and learning.*

*See you next week.*

*Regards,*

*Mercedes.*

The next time we met, Catherine thanked me for my 'lovely letter'. I wanted to know if anything had stood out in particular and she answered that the fact that I had taken the time to write it and that I had remembered her comment about the 'last 45 minutes'. I asked if she had found any of the questions interesting to think about. 'Not really', she responded with the blunt, honest and generous way of hers that I was starting to become more familiar with. So I ticked 'therapeutic documents' in my mental list as something that I needed to pay more attention to, and put it aside for the moment.

We went on to talk about some of the recent events with regard to her daughter's visit. Some of these had to do with changes in Catherine's initial considerations. She was still deeply concerned about the effect that the news could have on Mary to the point that she'd decided to go as a guy and be very gentle about letting her daughter know. My understanding is that this change came as a result of Catherine's skill of putting herself in someone else's position, in this case, her daughter's, and also from her knowledge about Mary, as a very sensitive young person.

Throughout our conversation, a much clearer and even detailed picture of the situation of breaking the news to Mary started to emerge. She started off with some rather broad categories – 'the right place' and 'the right time' – which were gradually unpacked, until we got to a fuller description of each of them. Catherine spoke of some of the conditions that would be important to consider: she said that the conversation with Mary would have to be in private and that they both needed to feel comfortable. She would have to wait until she found the right time and this had to do with both of them being relaxed, maybe sitting down. She said that being calm was going to be really important because she would then be in control and would have the space to think and, in turn, this would allow her to choose the words she would use. Later on she added the thought that it would be helpful if there could be someone there that could comfort Mary, someone that Mary was close to and felt comfortable with. Although Catherine had previously spoken of the close relationship between them, she said she knew that in that moment Mary would not find comfort with her but instead would feel distanced from her and that's why she'd wish for someone else to be there for Mary.

There were other conversations about family, work and 'breaking the news' that took place during that meeting. I had the opportunity to hear about Catherine's mother, who has passed away, and with whom Catherine had shared a close relationship. Actually, the thought of having someone to comfort Mary seemed to come from Catherine's consideration that it would be a good idea to think of her mother or evoke her presence while having the conversation with Mary. We also talked about other family members who Catherine also considered having a right to know about her decision and about her predictions of their reactions based on the knowledge that she has of them.

At the end of that session I asked Catherine how the conversation had gone for her. She said it was good, that it had been enlightening because now she had a clearer idea as to how to deal with the situation with her daughter. She also predicted that once having told Mary it would be easier to tell the rest of the people.

**Reflections**

Catherine's responses to both the document and the letter were very helpful in making me much more aware of the times when I went off by myself in the process, for example, when I suggested making a document which spoke about Catherine's history and her hopes. Now I have a different understanding of her hesitation to go this way (and by saying this I'm not implying that I can actually know what it was unless I asked her). My guess is, though, that her hesitation had to do with following my agenda, rather than her own. Catherine had said loud and clear from the beginning that she wanted to know about was *how* to tell her daughter rather than *what* to tell her, which was the aspect that the document focused on.

In looking back, I think that what got in the way of me being able to attend to Catherine's wish to address the issue of learning how to deal with that situation, had to do with the expectation that I would provide the answers or the information, in my role as a professional holding expert knowledge about relationships, interactions, families, communication, etc. What I forgot about at that moment, and was fortunately able to remember later on, was that very simple but fundamental idea that the people who consult therapists bring with them a life-long collection of knowledges and skills and that one of the purposes of narrative therapy is to generate conversations that will contribute to making those knowledges and skills more visible and more available for the person concerned. I believe that having this idea more present in my mind, would have allowed me to step out of what I now see as an apparent dilemma of having to perform the role of the expert in order to meet Catherine's expectations. Possibly it would also have prevented me from following my own agenda in my attempt to avoid that position.

With respect to the letter and to Catherine's response to it, I can think of a couple of things I'd do differently in the future. Firstly, I would discuss much more the purpose of the letter or document with the person so that it can become clearer how the document is going to be useful for them. I would also be more careful with the questions that I ask in these letters, trying to make sure they are not too broad so that they end up meaning very little or nothing to the person, as I think was the case with the questions I wrote in the letter to Catherine.

The previous thought leads to another consideration about what has been possible for me to become more aware of as a result of having these conversations with Catherine. Ways of 'scaffolding' conversations became more prominent not only as a thought but also as a practice. In the last meeting I began to pay a lot more attention to the kinds of questions that would be met by an inflexible 'I don't know' and the ones that would more likely engage Catherine with her own knowledges. For example, the question 'So, how does this 'right place' look like?' would more likely to be greeted with a response of 'I don't know', whereas 'Would it be a public space or would it be a place where you could be in private?' had a very definite answer that could be built upon. The idea of using a known situation as a reference, or a scaffold, to explore one that is unknown is something that I'm going to hold on to.

Finally, I believe I have now a different appreciation of not getting it right (I know that there is no such thing as the right question or the right conversation to be having with a client, but I still cannot get completely rid of the idea). In my nicest thoughts, mistakes represent lost opportunities. Yet, the opposite seems to be true in this case because I don't think I would have been reflecting in this way about my work if everything had gone well and I'd felt comfortable with what I did. I guess that alongside the realisation and my acceptance that mistakes will occur, I'm also committing to a more conscious practice, one that also acknowledges the contributions that people like Catherine make to giving life and shape to my work.

# 29

# A reflection from a transgender perspective

by

Esben Esther Pirelli Benestad

Let me begin with a general reflection about transgender people and therapy. Therapists' first encounters with transgendered people often pose unfamiliar challenges. At times it seems as if the transgendered individual becomes the practised professional, and the therapist becomes the client. My advice to other transgendered people in this position is to let the therapist pay for the consultations until she or he is sufficiently comfortable with transgender issues to activate her or his therapeutic skills! This, of course, is neither easy nor common, but is best accomplished, I believe, in an atmosphere where the therapist openly admits to her/his shortcomings on the issues of transgenderism. I believe that the original client should be given the choice of another and more transgender skilled therapist if such is available. If not, the challenge rests, as I have already mentioned, with the therapist's ability to learn from the client's insights.

The story described by Mercedes, to my ear, is of a process in which Catherine informs Mercedes through her transgendered story or narrative. Mercedes is temporarily lost before the challenge of how to assist Catherine inform her daughter, and then regains her skills in ways that are helpful to Catherine. I see no mistake done, besides the fact that Mercedes did not, it seems, take into consideration that she herself probably needed some time to process Catherine's story, before she could become therapeutically 'effective'.

In my experience, there is no right time or place for the sort of conversations that need to occur between Catherine and her daughter. It can be quite hard, even for a loving daughter, to be in the same room with her female father at the time of the first revelation. Sometimes there are bursts of anger, fear and/or hatred, although this is not common. The idea of her daughter having some other loved person with her, seems a good one. If this person was comfortable with Catherine's transgenderism, he or she could perhaps 'rejoice' with Mary on the concept of her father's trust and openness, and also contain possible rejecting reactions.

The greatest insights to the question of how to break news like this are within transgendered communities where such issues have been dealt with for ages. Significantly, in the story told by Mercedes, the 'solutions' were found within Catherine's own experiences in telling others about her situation. There is generally a tendency to imagine negative reactions to the presence of transgenderism in fathers, mothers, sisters or brothers. These imaginings very often represent internal catastrophes that actually very seldom materialise. This insight from the transgender community may soothe the therapeutic process of the client on her/his way to family revelations.

# PART EIGHT

# Complexities of culture, sexuality and spirituality

*Featuring African American, Egyptian, Australian and Jewish Israeli perspectives, this final section of the book explores the realm of culture, spirituality and sexuality.*

*These seem some of the most complex issues of all. One profoundly significant aspect of the gay and lesbian liberation movement has been a move towards developing a cross-cultural lesbian and gay consciousness – the development of a rainbow flag proudly symbolising a global queer community. Those with no voice in their families or communities can gather under this rainbow flag.*

*At the same time, however, the lesbian, gay, bisexual, transgender community is being continually challenged from within to look at and question how its assumptions and ways of being have been shaped largely by white western values. After all, the origins of the 'queer liberation movement' are routinely traced to Stonewall in New York City.*

*As the interviews and papers in the following section describe, these broader considerations of culture have very real effects on people's lives. They also generate profound dilemmas.*

*This is true in the personal as well as in the professional realm. For instance, here at Dulwich Centre Publications, we publish articles and books and organise conferences. We are a largely Anglo-Australian organisation which has a significant history of partnership with lesbian, gay, bisexual and transgender colleagues. Aspects of our work also involve partnerships across cultures (with Indigenous Australian, Jewish, Arab, Asian, and African colleagues), and across religions (including Christian, Muslim, Indigenous, and Judaism).*

*When issues relating to the intersection of culture and sexuality arise it can be extremely complex. This following section is dedicated to these complexities in the hope that further conversations can be shared about them.*

*As Moneira, a young Arab lesbian woman, asks in the first interview in this section, 'How can members of dominant cultural groups honour the struggle of gay, lesbian, bisexual and transgender people of every culture* and *respect the cultures from which they come?'*

*The last paper in this section is by Claire Ralfs and is entitled 'Who am I? Who are my people? And where do I belong?'. This paper, which is an exploration of lesbian feminist spirituality, was originally spoken in a plenary session at one of our conferences. We invited Claire to give this talk because the three largest world religions – Christianity, Judaism and Islam – have all played significant roles in justifying homophobia.*

*At times we have felt confused and saddened about the dilemmas involved in thinking through and responding to the intersection of culture and sexuality. At the same time, as we as members of dominant cultural groups try to face the implications of colonisation and racism, these issues seem of the utmost importance. We hope that the papers and interviews in this section contribute to further conversations, and we hope you, the reader, will be a part of them.*

# 30

# A woman of culture

## Negotiating Arabic and lesbian identity

an interview with

Moneira

*Moneira lives in Melbourne where she works in a young women's service. In this short interview she articulates some of the complexities of negotiating Arabic and lesbian identities. Moneira can be contacted c/o Dulwich Centre Publications. This interview was conducted over the phone by Claire Ralfs.*

*Within gay and lesbian contexts in Australia, there are strong notions about being 'out and proud'. How do these fit with your Arabic community context?*

They don't fit at all! For a whole range of reasons, I'm not 'out and proud' in the Arabic community. Far from it, I take care so that members of the Arabic community do not think I am lesbian. I take care with how I dress and how I act. Being lesbian is a significant part of my identity, and I have some sadness that I can't share this realm of my life with many of the people whom I love. Perhaps most sadly, when I've had partners, I haven't been able to take them home, and I know how much my mum loves feeding another person.

*It sounds like you know the Arab community would not be very receptive to your lesbian identity, what about the other way around...can you say a bit about your experience of being Arabic within the lesbian community? How is your Arabic identity received in that realm?*

I've been out in the lesbian community for three years now. Going into the lesbian community at first reminded me of when I began university. Back then, I was a young woman from the western suburbs going to Melbourne University, moving from a largely working class world to a place of the 'establishment'. It was quite an experience meeting people from different classes, different backgrounds. There were very few Arabs and not many others from non-Anglo cultures. I found the same thing going into the lesbian community. I had thought it would be a welcoming place, I guess that was naivety. I actually found it quite alienating. There are so many ways of being in the lesbian community that I find make me feel lonely, isolated and cold.

A part of this is due to the fact that my Arabic culture and heritage is never acknowledged or recognised within the lesbian community unless I draw attention to it. There are only a few lesbians I know with whom I can talk about being an Arab person. Well, it's a bit more complex than that because there are other lesbian Arabs in Melbourne but they make up almost a separate community and I've never really been into segregation. It's hard to find a balance and a place to be.

It's also tricky because within the lesbian community, being out and visible is a basis for connection. As I am not out within the Arab community it makes connections with other lesbians more complex.

*We have talked before about you being a woman of culture, and that there are particular practices of culture that are not well understood within the lesbian community. I wonder if you can talk a little bit more about this ...*

Well, I'm 30 years old and I am not 'out' as a lesbian to my parents. That is perhaps the biggest gap between Arabic culture and the Anglo world. The majority of the lesbian community would be very negative about my decision not to tell my parents. They would be quick to make judgments. But I have my reasons, and many of these are cultural. It wouldn't work for me in my community to be a visible lesbian.

Some of this is because of the homophobia of the Arab community which would be directed not only towards me but towards my family. As a political left wing lesbian Arab woman, various Anglo women tell me that I have a great opportunity to be out and lead the way in my community. Perhaps this is true, but I don't believe it is their place to make this judgment. They have no idea what the consequences would be for my life or my family.

Coming out for Anglo lesbians is very different than for Arab lesbians. Many people of Arab communities have recently migrated to this country. They are here without the supports they would have in their homeland. Many families have made great sacrifices for their children to be here. Many of the countries from where they come are very poor. All of these things shape the responses that families make to young Arab people when they come out. It is not a simple situation. There can be violence. And people from many Arab countries are not used to the idea of being able to appeal to the Anti-Discrimination Board or other structures. I regularly work with Arab and Middle Eastern women who are running away from home and I know that there are not support services that can realistically assist them. I know this because I work in the area.

There is an enormous amount of privilege that influences the views and understandings held by the Anglo lesbian community. I appreciate this privilege. I feel incredibly privileged to be living the sort of life I am in this country. I think of my cousins in Egypt who don't have the sorts of rights and opportunities that I have here. Neither did my parents. My father always used to say to me, don't ever take it for granted what this country has given us. As an Arab lesbian I don't take anything here for granted. I live with considerable privilege.

*Can you tell me about some of the things that have assisted you to live a life as a lesbian Arab woman?*

Like many people, I needed to overcome the shame that is caused by homophobia, and this took quite a long time. I guess this involved a process of accepting of who I was and wanted to be. Coming to know other lesbians who were not ashamed made a difference. A lesbian colleague that I work with was particularly supportive, we would laugh together and there was something about joining in laughter about all that we as lesbians have to contend with that was really helpful.

But it was actually when I was travelling that I fully came to terms with my sexuality. I returned to Egypt and was smoking a pipe one day at a coffee shop with my cousin when I told her I was a lesbian. She had the best reaction. She said, 'I'm really shocked, but then again I'm not'. This was the same reaction my brother had. They also both said in the same breath, 'You know you can never tell your family.' And I said, 'Yeah, I know.' But I had told them and they are family too. My cousin and I shared a bed for the three months after I told her and so she wasn't at all disturbed by it. I experienced her as very accepting. Having my brother know is excellent. When I spend time with him, I feel complete, I am myself. He is family and he knows who I am. All his friends know as well and they ask me questions, it's quite funny. So there are pockets of acceptance within my community through my brother and my cousin in Egypt. Maybe there will be one or two of my cousins here in Australia who will also be safe options in the future.

*This is really interesting to me. Rather than the 'out and proud' ethic of the (mainly Anglo) lesbian community, you seem to be living by a different ethic. You've clearly taken risks to talk to people from your Arabic community about your lesbian identity, but you are clear that it is not appropriate to tell others in your family. Can you tell me more about this different way of operating... is it linked in any way to Arabic culture?*

If I was to tell my mother that I am a lesbian it would break her heart. It would cause her extreme pain and difficulty in her community. She is already going through a very difficult time having lost my dad relatively recently. There is no way I am going to break my mother's heart. If that means I have to adjust my life accordingly, then I am willing to do that. Within the Anglo lesbian world there it little respect for this, it is often seen as the coward's way out. But I do not see it this way.

As an Arabic person, I have what is both a burden and a privilege, a duty to honour my parents for as long as I live. All Arab people have this duty, both men and women. In Egypt this means one thing. In Australia, the generations struggle over what this duty means. In our family it has meant both generations meeting half way between the cultural ways of Egypt and the cultural ways of Australia. My parents met me half way – sure it was a bit of a struggle for a while, perhaps it took 24 years - but they met me half way, and I honour this. My parents migrated countries for my future and for my brother's future. They have done everything they can to make sure that we live happy and prosperous lives. They have made many contributions to my quality of life and my capacity to live a life of my choosing.

If I was living in Egypt, I'd probably be married with kids by now. And for the person I am today, that would be horrible! But here I am. I have my own place. I am a lesbian. I can do my own thing. Everything I have here is a privilege that has been granted to me by my parents. They've met me half way and I have a duty to them to do the same. To tell my mother I am lesbian is not meeting her half way. It would be to break her heart and that's something I am not going to do.

*I imagine that the ways in which you have lived within these different worlds has led to you to develop particular knowledges about identity, about life ... can you say a bit about this?*

One thing it has meant, is that I have developed a sense of clarity about what is fair and what is not fair. I have a sensitivity, interest and curiosity in fairness. I think this is because I have had to balance that in my own life for a long time. I've had to think through what Egyptian cultural practices I think are fair enough for me to engage with, and which Anglo cultural practices I think are fair to participate in. I've also witnessed up close, many different versions fairness, of pride and dignity. I think of my father when I mention these things. In my culture, pride and dignity are crucial concepts of identity. My father had very rich ways of understanding what it means to be treated fairly and to live a proud and dignified life.

*How do you think these special knowledges influence your work with young women?*

I think I had some sort of sensitivity to understanding what people can and can't do depending on their own context. For instance, I can see very clearly if someone is being setup to fail. I see the broader influences on people's lives and I'm also quick to look for cultural meanings where others might ignore them.

Recently, a group of professional women came out to talk to the young women at the youth service where I work. The way in which the meeting was set up meant that only the white young women felt comfortable to speak. There was a cultural gap in the protocols, but this was understood in a certain way by those who had come to visit. They though that these islander young women were gang members who were sticking together and not opening their mouths. Their silence was seen as a form of rebellion, but I could see quite clearly this wasn't the case.

Afterwards, when I spoke with the young women they said that they hadn't felt as if they the right to speak. In many cultures there are different understandings about when it is appropriate to speak and when it is not. These young women of culture were actually quite softly spoken and their actions had been completely misunderstood. They would need a context to be created in which they felt entitled to speak. These sorts of cultural misunderstandings happen all the time. I think because of my own experience I have a sensitivity to them.

*What advice would you give to other workers who are relating to Arab women, especially in relation to matters of sexuality?*

When I think about that question, it makes me wonder what would have been most helpful to me. You know, I reckon it would be great to receive some acknowledgment that it can be pretty tricky being both Arabic and lesbian! If there could be respect for what it takes to balance a life between Arabic identity and lesbian identity it would make it easier. It would make it easier if there was respect for the struggle, and also respect for Arab culture.

The homophobia in the Arab community that I mentioned earlier, is just one aspect of a huge culture. Like many cultures, my culture is homophobic. But my culture is also very loving and hospitable and caring. There are many beautiful aspects of being Arabic that I treasure.

We have a bond of family that I respect. No matter how low you get, there will always be people there for each other. We have ways of relating with food and celebrations that I delight in. And then there's the laughter...we can laugh for hours. My uncle makes up stories and we laugh. We sit around together and we all go out together. This is the beauty of living life through extended family relationships. There are also smaller traditions that are of both family history and cultural history. There is the giving of gifts, the rituals that bring with them a sense of belonging. There's a generosity and, of course, the language which holds its own meanings and metaphors and ways of understanding life. Then there is music...I could go on....I feel very privileged to live with all of this and more.

For workers who are relating to young lesbian Arabic women, I think it would be significant to acknowledge their struggle and to respect it, while at the same time respecting their culture. This is what would have meant a lot to me.

*At the moment there is considerable hostility being directed towards the Arab community in Australia – especially in relation to asylum seeker issues. How are you and others in your community managing to sustain life, and relationships and love and passion during these times?*

There are many different ways. With my close friends we try always to laugh, while in my work, it is taking action that sustains me. I am involved in a range of projects to try to address the effects of racism on young Arab people. Knowing that I do a good job at this is sustaining. I'm proud that I'm an Arabic woman who is living in Melbourne and who is a lesbian. It's made me strong and I know now that I will always land on my feet.

But perhaps what sustains me the most is knowing that I'm privileged. It humbles me when I get an email from my cousin who's been waiting for two and half years for a phone line. Knowing that I'm privileged sustains me, and it invites me to take action. No matter how difficult life can be here, it could be so much more difficult. Life is so much more difficult for other Arabs, for other women, for other lesbians. We must do something about this.

# 31

# A glimpse of the complexity of identity

by

Tikka Jan Wilson

*Can you perhaps say a little about how you understand the relationship between your experience as an African-American woman, as a person who has lived a life outside mainstream notions of sexual identity, and as someone who was adopted as a child? Are these different realms of experience somehow related to one another?*

These are interesting considerations. There is, to me, some connection between being adopted, being African-American and being a lesbian. I don't think lesbianism is any way an 'essential' part of me. Far from it, I think my lesbian identity has been shaped by all my experiences of life.

I felt very much an outsider within my adopted family. For whatever reason, I felt a fundamental difference from my parents. This wasn't due to race, they were black as well, but it may have been a part of my particular adoption experience, or it could have been age. Back then, you had to be pretty old to adopt a child. My parents came of age at the turn of WWI. I came of age in the 1960s. The distance between us could have been history. For whatever reason, I didn't feel I belonged to them.

This sense of not belonging was also influenced by the fact that my parents had grown up in the south of the US and had then migrated to the north. Due to this migration we lived without an extended family. As well, I grew up in a white neighbourhood. There were all sorts of dislocations and experiences of not really belonging, not only in relation to my immediate family, but to the community around us.

Then there were expectations about getting married and being sexual, and I found this all pretty complex. Heterosexual relationships were still starkly segregated. People didn't date across race lines very much in those days. So, I was clearly supposed to date and eventually marry another black person. The trouble was, these other black people were not around. I think that my early experiences of heterosexuality were quite fraught because of all of this. The only sort of relationship I had with young black men was through dating, and this influenced the shape of those relationships.

For me then, when I found a lesbian community, it was one of the first times I felt I could belong on my own merit. Although there were many problematic aspects of the relationship between black and white lesbians at that time (as there still are), there was also a sense of community across racial lines that I hadn't experienced as a heterosexual woman. While my attempts to negotiate heterosexual relationships had occurred in a starkly segregated context, the lesbian community of Boston in the 1970s was a community of people of different races who were coming together around sexuality.

I don't want to make it sound simplistic though. To be an African-American lesbian in the 1970s was to be seen as something of a 'race traitor'. This was the time of 'Black Power' and black consciousness and the role of black women was to support and stand in solidarity with black men. Homophobia has specific racial configurations and there were strong invitations to black women to relate to black men in certain ways at that time. Those invitations succeeded in making me feel some guilt, but the other black lesbians were helpful in articulating the sexism implicit in these ideas.

As an African-American, I know that my lesbianism was incredibly embarrassing for my parents, as I imagine children's homosexuality initially is for many parents of white children. Here again though, it made a difference that I had been adopted. For adopting parents, it's probably very weird to have a gay or lesbian child. Those questions about 'did I do something wrong' are perhaps even more difficult for adoptive parents. I suspect that there's some sort of gap between adoptive parents and their children that can make sexuality even more difficult to negotiate.

So yes, my experience of lesbianism, of being African-American and being adopted are certainly all inter-related. It's not really possible to understand them separately.

*Could you say some more about what it was about the lesbian community in Boston in the 1970s that enabled the sense of belonging that you mentioned? Were there certain community practices that made this more possible?*

Perhaps most significant was that the lesbians I hung out with did not expect me to be hyper feminine. I had always experienced femininity as a requirement to be stupid. If some guy said something that he felt was terribly smart and wonderful, and if I knew it was totally incorrect, then I was supposed to keep my mouth shut and pretend to be an idiot. For some reason this never fitted very well for me! Entering the lesbian community meant getting free of those expectations of femininity and this was a delight.

At the time I was working as a motion picture operator and the sexism was really profound. Yet with lesbians, it was perfectly fine to step outside of sex stereotyped occupations and ways of being and to be able to be proud of this rather than embarrassed by it. I was able to be athletic, to ride motorcycles and do other things that at that time were transgressive gender behaviour. In the 21st century all of this is totally unremarkable, but then it was significant and quite scary. Within the lesbian community these other, non-feminine ways of being women were all valued. It was an incredible relief.

Boston was a wonderful place to come out. There were many lesbian bars and it was so freeing to be able to go to a pub and not worry about men. I would never have just gone to a local heterosexual bar without a man in tow (or without being towed by a man!), but I was able to go to lesbian bars on my own and shoot a game of pool. It seems such a small pleasure looking back but it was significant then.

Most of the lesbian bars were mixed race and that was quite unusual in the US at that time. The gay and lesbian community was less segregated, differently segregated, and all these things were liberating.

I think from those times I could see that it was really possible for people who were very different to somehow negotiate those differences. Sure there would be difficulties and shouting matches, but it seemed possible. Everybody was trying and that was a real opening. It was a gift.

So too was the sense of belonging that I found there. To belong involves having a sense of community with other people whom you feel at some level you have a fundamental similarity too. That is what I did not have in my family or my neighbourhood. The lesbian community was where I felt that I could be comfortable, where things that I liked to do, other people liked to do. It's not that there weren't ways that we were expected to conform, there were, but they were just easier than what hyper femininity had expected of me. I felt cared for and at times there was a sense of belonging that was new to me. The things that hadn't been valued about me before, were now being valued, and that was precious.

But this was all a long time ago, culturally and historically. The seventies was a time of transition. People had always lived double lives around sexuality and now they were coming out. It was a slow transition. Not everyone just leaped out of the closet! But things have changed radically since the 1970s. Not least, I now live in Australia.

*Perhaps we could talk now about Australia. Can you say a little bit about what must have been a big transition moving from the US to this country?*

My experiences in relation to sexual identity and racial identity are very different here. Partly this is because I am a lot older, and my sexual identity is a lot less important to me now than it once was. It's just a part of my life now whereas in the period I was talking about before it was most of my life. My whole world was then structured around being lesbian and that is different now.

The other reason why issues of sexual identity are no longer as central to my life is because, at least in the circles in which I live, homophobia is no longer so rampant. At work, everyone knows that I am lesbian, as do the people with whom I generally mix. A lot has changed and so my life here in Australia is less centred around lesbian life, politics and identity.

The intersection of racism and homophobia is also different for me here. My experience of racism in this country is as someone who is marginal to the two fundamental axes of racism in Australia. These fundamental axes are between white people and Indigenous people, and between white people and Asian people. There are deep and significant histories in this country in relation to conquest, exploitation, exclusion and all the accompanying laws, emotions, fears, hatreds and self-hatreds. As an African-American I am on the margins of all of this. In fact, in this country, I am often located as an honorary white person. I get many of the privileges of being white, and often feel as if I am a not quite white person. Because of this I rarely experience the intersections of race and sexuality in the ways that I am sure Aboriginal and Asian lesbian women must experience here.

Still, the issues do come up. I am in a cross racial relationship with Manja Visschedijk, who immigrated to Australia from Holland as a child. There have certainly been times, such as when we have been trying to rent a place to live, when the intersections of homophobia and racism have been vividly clear. Actually, though, in our relationship, most of our discussions are about different experiences of race and class.

*Can you say a little more about this?*

Where Manja is from a working-class immigrant background, I am from a middle-class/professional black background. Now in the US, there is a considerable debate about class amongst African-Americans, and an acknowledgement of how class shapes black experience. But in the 1960s, the real economic differences between the black middle-class and the black working-class were somehow hidden or buried under a sense of being united in the civil rights movement. Then, as now, class was complicated by race – the economic differences between black middle-class life opportunities and white middle-class life opportunities were stark.

I bring these histories into all the discussions that Manja and I have about class. Actually, for Manja, what stands out about me is class rather than race. I think this is complex though because I believe Manja associates being middle-class with being white! We can have big misunderstandings about the connections between race and class! I see her as having considerable race privilege (about which she would agree) and she would see that I have considerable class privilege (about which I agree).

While this can lead to plenty of arguments, it can also lead to intriguing conversations. A classic example was when we were driving together and saw a car broken down on the side of the road and three or four white men gesturing for help. Manja read their class position as being working-class and wanted to stop and help them. I read their race position and there was no way I was going to stop for white men on the side of a road! It was very interesting how strong both of our responses were. Where I saw them as a very real threat, Manja saw them as people like her. It was absolutely fascinating! After a heated discussion we kept going. At least we could agree on the gender issue, that perhaps as two lesbian women stopping for four men wasn't so wise and that we could leave it to someone else this time.

What's also significant is that we are both migrants. I have no idea of what the Australian culture was like that Manja grew up in (after they moved from the Netherlands) and she has no idea of the intricacies of US culture. This all leads to a lot of interesting scenarios!

*Knowing both you and Manja, I can imagine how you would put your different views of the world to great use ...*

It's certainly been an eye-opener for both of us. There are so many areas in which our assumptions about life and how we see the world vary. We even interpret the same words differently. We come from different places and we can help to make sense of each other's experiences of life. This is pretty interesting. Where it becomes most powerful is when we can observe the different ways in which people relate to us.

There are so many minute practices of life in this culture that otherwise I would have never known about. To be able to experience these things together, differently, and then talk with each other about it brings a richness to the relationship and also to life itself. We're always learning from the other's perspective.

*Thanks Tikka. I've no doubt that others will really enjoy learning from your perspective as they read this interview.*

# 32

# An open house in the Holy City

from an interview with

## Jerry Levinson

*Jerry lives and works in Israel and is the Co-Founder and Chair of The Open House – Gay, Lesbian, Bisexual and Transgender Community Centre in Jerusalem, Israel.*

I was almost 18 when I came to Israel in 1969. In some ways I was running away from being gay in US and in those younger years I tried to do what those around me did – I went out with girlfriends, I acted straight, even went to therapy in attempt to cover up a sexuality which intimidated me. As I grew older this began to change and by the time I was forty, not only was I out as a gay man but I came to see that if we as gay, lesbian, bisexual, transgender people don't make changes to this world then no one else is going to do it for us.

This newfound determination led me to volunteer on a gay support hotline and later to become a supervisor for counsellors for a gay youth support group in Tel Aviv. Then, seven years ago, a group of lesbian and gay activists came together here in Jerusalem to try and determine what sort of service we would like to see exist to serve the local gay, lesbian, bisexual, transgender community.

Jerusalem is a unique city in Israel and in the world. It is the meeting place of three world religions (all of which are powerfully homophobic) and it is a city of enormously diverse cultural and religious communities. There are Arab Christians and Arab Muslims as well as Jewish Israelis some of whom hail from other countries including Ethiopia, Russia and other Middle Eastern countries. There are secular Jews and there are very large orthodox and ultra orthodox religious communities. The lives of these different cultural and religious groups barely touch one another, let alone overlap, except perhaps in downtown Jerusalem when people come together to shop. It is, quite simply, an extraordinary city.

This separation of communities has many implications. Within each cultural and religious community there is of course an invisible lesbian and gay sub-community. But until recently, these sub-communities did not know of each others' existence.

Then, over coffee and apple cake one day, we decided that Jerusalem deserved a gay and lesbian community centre – and the Open House was born. We have existed now for five years and over that time have experienced meteoric growth not only in terms of what we are offering, but also in terms of a sense of hopefulness.

**Religion and sexuality**

One of the communities that has been involved in the growth of the Open House has been the Jewish religious and orthodox communities. We are currently linked with four orthodox and ultra-orthodox self-help support groups. While they do not meet at the Open House, they are associated with us and we refer them potential members. We have also established an open Jewish learning forum – a Beit Midrash – for the study of religious texts that pertain to sexuality, homosexuality, and pluralism within Judaism. This provides the opportunity for people to congregate in a framework of study.

At times, we have also held public symposia on religion and homosexuality. After one of these lectures a young orthodox man approached to thank me for 'saving his life'. While I tried to articulate that this was not necessary, and that I barely knew him, he was insistent. He described how he had been completely ostracised by his family and evicted from his home when he came out as gay. His entire social links were broken. He articulated how he was seen as anathema to his community and how the youth support group at the Open House was all that enabled him to hold onto hope during this crisis.

This young man's experience, while perhaps more extreme than some, is a commonly heard story at the Open House from young men of all three of the world religions that meet in Jerusalem. All three religions – Judaism, Christianity and Islam – are profoundly homophobic. I am reminded of a Muslim young man who came to see us over a year ago. After he had come out to his family, while he has not been ostracised, he has instead been subjected to physical beatings in his home because he is gay. He has also had imposed upon him a 6pm curfew so that he doesn't go out and look for men. Young Arab men and women in Jerusalem do not leave their family home until they are married. This young man is in a terrible bind.

People who feel strong identification with religious teachings (Christian, Muslim or Judaism) often find particular difficulty in integrating their religious identity with their sexual orientation. What we try to provide through our support groups is a way to integrate these identities to the extent that this is possible. Acknowledging that there is a conflict between these identities and trying to build a bridge and offer company in the process seems to make a considerable difference to what is a very complex situation.

A recent film, 'Trembling before G-D' is playing a significant part in enabling different conversations around these issues. Rabbi Steve Greenberg, who used to facilitate our Beit Midrash, is currently touring the world with this film which has already been in cinemas here in Israel and will soon be shown on television. It's an inspiring film about the experience of homosexuality within orthodox Jewish religious communities in Israel, Great Britain and the USA. It constitutes an extremely valuable tool in describing the effects of stigma on people's lives and ways of talking across differences.

Most ultra orthodox people whom we have contact with do not physically come to the Open House – although some do and spend time in our library. Most do not wish to visit the building, both because of the fear of being seen but also because they are worried that outsiders will try to proselytise them away from their religion. We are committed to trying to assist lesbian, gay, bisexual, transgender people of all communities and religions to find peace with their identities. This involves care and thoughtfulness, not proselytising.

## Questions of culture

The experience of people within different cultural groupings is also very complex. For instance, within the Jewish Ethiopian community here in Jerusalem there are no visible lesbian, gay, bisexual or transgender people. In this community there is tremendous stigma associated with these identities and at the same time a tremendous importance placed on community cohesion. To be identified as homosexual would be to face ostracism and this, literally, is a fate worse than death for people of this community.

In the Jewish Russian community, however, there are now young Russians who are changing this particular community's views. When the older Russians first immigrated in the 1980s they came from a country in which homosexuality was an 'unmentionable'. While much has changed in Russia since then, the older Russians have not witnessed this and this has consequences here. The Russian press in Israel, for example, is very homophobic. But the younger generation is making changes.

In the Arab communities too, both Christian and Muslim, homosexuality is seen as unacceptable. There are no openly 'out' lesbian Arabs in Israel. There are probably only 50 'out' Arab gay men, many of whom are from relatively privileged families and have spent time outside the country studying in Europe.

Homophobia has a different face depending on the particular community – sometimes homophobia takes the shape of religious based oppression, other times societal stigma. Whatever its face, it has tremendous effects on the individuals of each community.

## What we are doing

Here at the Open House all of our work has a dual purpose. Firstly, to empower the gay, lesbian, bisexual, transgender community in Jerusalem, many of whom are closeted and who live life behind closed doors for fear of persecution. And secondly, to change the broader attitudes that are currently affecting this invisible community. Whether we are talking in schools, opening an anonymous AIDS testing unit, training youth workers or offering self-help groups, crisis counselling and referrals, we are always thinking of these two purposes, to empower the community and to change the broader attitudes.

Many people who live in Jerusalem are poor and most cannot afford therapy. One of the first things we did was to set up a group of lesbian and gay therapists, social workers and psychologists with the aim of being able to provide subsidised therapy. At the moment we cannot afford to provide long-term counselling but we do offer crisis intervention and short term therapy and provide referrals where required.

A year ago we also formed a national association of gay, lesbian, bisexual and transgender psychotherapists, social workers, art therapists and psychiatrists. As yet we don't have any psychiatrists as members, and I think this is due to the stigma within that community. We do however have over 90 members and have established peer supervision groups in both Tel Aviv and Jerusalem.

We are very proud of what is being achieved here. While Stonewall occurred in 1969, and some looking on from outside may believe that our work is a little behind the times, we know that we're just starting to make inroads in a city where the context is so very different than pretty much anywhere else. Even before the recent Intifada began, Jerusalem has always been segregated. The different cultural and religious communities here are relatively isolated from one another.

The Open House is one of the very few institutions that is providing an opportunity for people from different cultural and religious groups to come together, to mix, to talk and to share experiences. Lesbian, gay, bisexual and transgender people from all of the different communities are contacting each other through the Open House. This provides me with considerable hope. I do not believe this is happening in the same way elsewhere in the city or in the country at this time for that matter. There is close collaboration here between lesbian women and gay men – we have a majority of women on our board. There is an Arab Muslim on our board. There are transgender people integrating more and more throughout our organisation. There are straight people as volunteers and as employees. There is an Arab population co-ordinator. There are religious and non-religious people involved in all aspects of our work. And representatives from many of the different cultural communities pass through our doors.

In a way, we're trying to learn how to speak a different language. A language that does not categorise each other into stigmatised and non-stigmatised groupings. It sounds simple when I say it like that, but it is a very complex and difficult matter. Tolerance, pluralism and accepting each others' differences sound as if they should be easy, but they are not. What gives me hope is when I see small movement within these processes. I'm happy that the Open House is being able to make changes to individual people's lives. I see these changes on people's faces in workshops and lectures, I see change occurring in therapy sessions, in self-help groups, and we will see it when we walk down the streets of Jerusalem on our first Pride march next month. There are bound to be many difficulties placed in our way between now and then but we will be marching on June 7th.

Jerusalem is an extraordinary city, and the Open House an extraordinary institution with a compelling message for all: that mutual tolerance and multi-culturalism can be much more than slogans, that oppressed minorities such as the lesbian, gay, bisexual and transgender community can do much to affect stigmatic social norms and attitudes in their struggle to achieve liberation, and that this process can have a profound effect in transforming individual lives in the direction of greater empowerment, peace of mind and self-integration. I wish you could all be here to march with us on June 7th.

# 33

# 'Trembling before G-D'

a reflection by

## Margaret Newmark

*Margaret Newmark is a straight-talking straight family therapist in private practice in New York City, who kindly agreed to write this reflection of* Trembling before G-D.

*Trembling before G-D* is a documentary film about gay people caught between the every day reality of their lives and the beliefs and practices of Orthodox Judaism. Made in Israel by Sandi Simcha Dubowski, it follows the testing of faith of men and women as they confront the demand by the religion they love that they deny the way they love. The film follows several people as they struggle to maintain their integrity. The voicing of these struggles is woven together with interviews with rabbis, scenes of Orthodox Jewish men praying, playing and studying together, and with glimpses of the practices of fai  n the daily lives of the gay people who are excluded from that society.

As I try to describe this film I realise once again how carefully the director has preserved the complexities of the dilemma so that the audience can experience them without interference from him. Juxtaposing the theological positions of the rabbi and their translation into practice, Dubowski seems to create a tension between intellectual understanding and emotional understanding that kept me from escaping into easy judgements.

Why did I insist on seeing this movie, standing in line on a cold, windy night? Why do I keep returning to it in my mind? Having no religious training, I have been a religion groupie since I was a small child going to church with my friend Cynthia as she made her novena, going once to Hebrew school with the children across the street, singing in the children's choir of the Episcopal church. As a teenager I read everything I could find about Catholic monastic and convent life. I knew I was Jewish because my aunt told me when I was seven that I was lucky: if my birthday had fallen on Yom Kippur, I couldn't have had any cake. That was the beginning and the end of my Jewish education.

The fascination with religion and particularly with the clash between the dictates of faith and real life abides. But seeing this film is the first time I have been about to sympathise emotionally as well as intellectually with that struggle in Judaism. The scenes of Orthodox men in the synagogue invited me into the warmth and security and celebration of their relationship to each other and to G-D, just as Rumer Godden invites you into the convent in 'This House of Brede' (1991). The scenes of Orthodox gay women preparing for the Sabbath and lighting candles gave me the chance to feel

The dailiness of their personal relationship to faith through religious practice. These women would be excluded from direct participation in the rituals of the synagogue no matter what their sexual orientation; the gay men are excluded only because of their sexual orientation; and both feel the loss of community full force.

Although I had read many descriptions from many religions, I had never literally seen what it might mean for a believer to be excluded from the practice of belief, or that the practice made the community, not the shared belief per se. Of course, this is the loss of what one might call 'public' community. 'Private' community, of family, friends and partners remains. Does it make up for the loss? What are the lonelinesses of the people who are cut off from their families and public worship, and of people who don't even have partners? How then do you keep your faith in yourself when you are being told you are sinning, and when you are alone and sinning? This film respectfully pulls you into the heart of these questions.

# 34

# Who am I? Who are my people? And where do I belong?[1]

by

Claire Ralfs

I wish to acknowledge that I am on Kaurna Land[1] and that I speak in the presence of many indigenous people and people from other cultures.

In being asked to speak about spirituality I have had to think deeply about my relationship to belief and faith. I have had to consider as a white, middle-class lesbian woman, what place if any spirituality has in my life. I guess I'm here to say that spirituality, faith and belief has a significant part of my life, in spite of my lack of participation within organised or defined religion.

I am a daughter of two ex-Salvation Army parents. Their marriage was the opportunity for both my parents to flee from the constraints and regulations of the Salvation Army. They made a brief attempt to insist their children go to the local Sunday school, but I was the fourth child and they had abandoned the project by the time I was old enough to attend. Consequently I am untrained in the religion of Christianity or any other religion.

I am the product of the secular, capitalist society that has turned ritual and spirituality into an orgy of consumerism and commercialism. Finding my way to spirituality within this context is not simple.

The absence of organised religion is easily replaced by the God of money with its daily and weekly consumer rituals. Retail therapy is widely practiced as an effective relief from all sorts of modern ailments. However, its benefits are usually short-lived and ongoing shopping expeditions are generally required. This tends to lead to unwanted side effects such as debt and unwanted junk that we thought we needed. I have found the temple of consumption to be very alluring but rarely truly satisfying.

It has been through the challenges from indigenous women that I have been able to explore more satisfying strategies to create ritual and meaning in my life. Alternatives to ongoing consumption as a way of experiencing the world around me have led me into relationships of belonging to my community and the environment I live in. From this belonging, faith, purpose and meaning have been able to unfold for me. This meaning or purpose is not fixed or definitive but it is a base, a foundation from which I grow and live and will ultimately die.

The beginning of this journey was from a series of questions asked of me by Kaurna women in the early 80s. These questions were: 'Who are you? Who are your people? And where do you belong?'. These questions profoundly affected me. The obvious answer: white middle-class lesbian, fourth child, born in Melbourne, seemed very superficial. Yet in truth I could not name much more at the time.

What I began to be able to understand and answer first was that I was a tenant in Australia. I live here and enjoy its beauties, its freedoms, its enormous skies and its wealth, and I do all this on Aboriginal Land. I am a tenant.

Realising this really helped my sense of belonging. I had a good understanding of how to be a good and respectful tenant. The responsibilities and requirements of 'paying the rent' fitted my cultural framework perfectly. As I said earlier, the temple of consumption knows lots about paying bills.

This recognition of my relationship to this land as a tenant has been an important place from which to develop my understanding of myself and my cultural heritage. An essential element of these early learnings was being able to distinguish between what is my personal heritage, what is my collective cultural heritage, and what is someone else's cultural heritage. These distinctions have served me well in building respectful relationships that seek to honour the beliefs and rituals that fall outside my experiences.

This is about learning from other cultures. Learning from other cultures and religions rather than appropriating or souveniring other cultures has also been a central lesson in this journey. This is not an easy lesson when my collective cultural heritage of centuries of invasion and appropriation of a whole host of different cultures. Regularly noticing where the rituals are drawn from helps me to honour the traditions that have shaped me and also draws me into relationships with others across time and context.

Creating rituals that facilitate connectedness helps me to answer the questions: Who am I? Who are my people? And where do I belong?

What I can now say about myself is very different from when I was first asked these questions seventeen years ago. I know so much more about my heritage of being a lesbian and the world of silences and secret codes and intense belonging.

I know the different silences of being a relinquishing mother and the heritage of living outside the mainstream structures of our social arrangements. I continually learn about the interplay in my own life, between marginalisation and mainstream privilege.

The rituals of birthdays, summer solstice, our local community dinners and my team meetings all provide an antidote to the sense of isolation that can be generated through being different. One of the oldest rituals in my life is summer solstice. This pagan ritual resurrected through feminism is celebrated by my community through sharing our reflections of the year passed and hopes for the coming year. It also includes a present-giving ceremony in which everyone has chosen a name from a hat three months prior and we each make our person a present. We are not allowed to buy a present. Every year this ritual so close to the chaos of western commercial Christmas feels like a burden. The effort of making presents and supporting children to make presents seems like so much work. However, each year when we give our presents and share our year we all know we'll be doing it next year.

From our solstice ritual we have given meaning to the art and joy of giving as opposed to consuming. I have a wonderful collection of t-shirts with children's paintings on them, home made calendars and painted boxes made by children and adults, each of them a delight to receive and each coming to me with a story about why they were made for me. I draw strength from the belonging these communal rituals mark and make visible to all of us who participate.

Not all my rituals are communal. Many are solitary – sitting with chooks, watching the sun set, noticing the change in season, visiting the same piece of bush or same bit of beach just to notice the different ways the passage of time is experienced. Doing these things helps me to be in the moment, in my life, to notice me and who I am. And they remind me that I am part of much bigger life cycle that my own life.

From these rituals I am acutely aware of the urgent need for healing the earth. Learning to caretake the environment is a big task that will require the collective efforts of us all. We need to create some shared commitment to protecting and caring for our shared environment. This is a huge task and one we need to get on with now not later. For me this translates into the development of daily skills in caring. Learning to be carers is another major challenge to the practices of consumption and throw away culture.

Within our community caring is about learning to relate well. To address our struggles and conflicts with each other in ways that move us closer rather than further apart. It also means not living within a nuclear family construct. This recently involved two parents within our community resigning from their struggles with their daughter over homework. Louise and Simon, Anna's parents, for a long time had a big struggle with getting the homework done. It wasn't working and they were feeling pretty bad with each other. Through our community and our caring for each other it became obvious that Anna still needed help with her homework but maybe not her parents' help. So our household – six doors down from theirs – is now responsible for helping Anna with her homework. And Louise and Simon have been able to resign from this struggle. They are now able to put much more effort into having a good time with Anna, free of the anguish of this fight. And our household is now where Anna visits her Homework Aunties every Monday night and we take pleasure in finding her books and giving her Homework Auntie advise.

Within our community, through getting better at caring for each other, we are creating daily rituals of respect and love.

From this place it is much easier to value the diversity of people, particularly in their ways of making meaning in their worlds. My rituals are so new and my meanings are often fragile and unclear, however, this is the world I am in – where the organised religions and spiritualities are either not intact or do not help me as a white middle-class, lesbian woman to make sense of the world

In developing this speech and exploring how spirituality expresses itself in my life I have come to realise that my faith and hope for the future is enriched by my regular spiritual practices of continually finding answers to the questions: Who am I? Who are my people? And where do I belong?

Thank you for listening.

## Note

1. The Kaurna people are the traditional custodians of the land on which the city of Adelaide now stands. In Australia, it is becoming customary, as a sign of respect, to acknowledge the Indigenous Australian peoples of the land prior to speaking at a formal event like a conference.

# Contributors

## Christopher Behan & James Light

Christopher and James live in Portland, Maine, USA, and can be contacted c/o cbehan@sweetser.org Christopher can also be contacted c/o The Family Institute of Maine, 65 West Commercial Street, Portland, ME, USA

## Esben Esther Pirelli Benestad

Esben Esther works in Grimstad MPAT – Institute on the southern coast of Norway. In addition to her/his transgender experiences, she/he is a medical doctor, family therapist and sexologist. Esben Esther can be contacted c/o Grimstad MPAT-Institute, Storgaten 40/42, 4876 Grimstad, Norway. Tel: 47 37 258100, Fax 47 37 258105, Email: esben.esther@sexologi.com

## Paul Browde & Murray Nossel

Paul and Murray both live and work in New York City and can be contacted c/o narativ inc., 878 West End Avenue #5B, New York City NY 10025, USA. Murray's email address is: mln6@columbia.edu Paul's email address is: pbrowde@hotmail.com

## David Denborough

David works as staff writer at Dulwich Centre Publications

## Daphne Hewson

Daphne lives and works in Sydney, and can be contacted c/o School of Behavioural Sciences, Macquarie University, Nth Ryde NSW 2109, Australia

## Zoy Kazan

Zoy lives and works in California and can be contacted c/o www.narrativetherapy.org

## Joan Laird & Ann Hartman

Joan and Ann live in rural Massachusetts, and can be contacted via email at (Ann) Lahart7894@aol.com (Joan) joanlaird@aol.com

## Jerry Levinson

Jerry lives and works in Israel and is the Co-Founder and Chair of The Open House – Gay, Lesbian, Bisexual and Transgender Community Centre in Jerusalem, Israel. Web: gay.org.il/joh Email: jerry@joh.gay.org.il

## Bill Logan

Bill lives and works in New Zealand and can be contacted c/o Dulwich Centre Publications.

## Mercedes Martinez

Mercedes is a young Mexican psychologist who moved to Australia in 2000 for one year to study narrative therapy at Dulwich Centre. Mercedes lives and works in Mexico city where she can be contacted c/o: mmtzc@hotmail.com

## *Chris McLean*

Chris lives in Adelaide, Australia, and can be contacted c/o Dulwich Centre Publications.

## *Frann Michel*

Frann works at the Dept of English at Willamette University, where she can be contacted c/o 900 State St, Salem OR 97301, USA.

## *Moneira*

Moneira lives and works in Melbourne, Australia, and can be contacted c/o Dulwich Centre Publications.

## *Margaret Newmark*

Margaret is a straight-talking straight family therapist in private practice in New York City, who kindly agreed to write this reflection of Trembling before G-D. Margaret can be contacted c/o 865 West End Avenue, #10A, New York NY 10025, USA.

## *Patrick O'Leary*

Patrick lives and works in Adelaide, Australia, and can be contacted c/o Dulwich Centre Publications.

## *Amy Ralfs*

Amy lives in Adelaide, Australia, where she is currently studying at university, and can be contacted c/o Dulwich Centre Publications.

## *Claire Ralfs*

Claire Ralfs lives and works in Adelaide, Australia, and can be contacted c/o Dulwich Centre Publications.

## Jane Speedy

Jane lives and works in Bristol, England, and can be contacted c/o Jane.Speedy@Bristol.ac.uk

## Suzy Stiles

Suzy lives and works in Adelaide, Australia, and can be contacted c/o Dulwich Centre Publications.

## Mark Trudinger

Mark lives and works in Brisbane, Australia, and can be contacted c/o PO Box 5375, West End QLD 4101, Australia.

## Manja Visschedijk

Manja works at Relationships Australia in Adelaide, South Australia, and can be contacted c/o: manjaviss@yahoo.com

## Tikka Wilson

Tikka lives and works in Canberra, Australia, and can be contacted c/o: tikkaw2000@aol.com

# Information about the papers

## Part One

All the papers in Part One were spoken in a plenary session on 'Celebrating alternative families' at Dulwich Centre Publications' International Narrative Therapy & Community Work Conference which was held in Adelaide in February 2001, and were first published in *Dulwich Centre Journal* 2001 No.1. Except Amy's story which was first published in *Dulwich Centre Journal* 1995 Nos.2&3 'Schooling & education: Exploring new possibilities'; and 'Amy Ralfs' story' by Amy Ralfs which was first published in the book entitled Narrative Therapy & Community Work: A conference collection (1999, Dulwich Centre Publications).

## Part Two

'Heterosexual dominance in the world of therapy?' by Daphne Hewson was first published in *Dulwich Centre Journal,* 1993 No.2.

'The power of language' by Suzy Stiles and 'Speaking out from the dominant position' by Chris McLean were first published in *Comment,* 1995 No.2.

'Who Cares? Institutional barriers to health care for lesbian, gay and bisexual persons', by Michele J. Eliason, a review by David Denborough, was first published in *Gecko,* 1999 No.1

## Part Three

This paper was first published in *Dulwich Centre Journal*, 2000 Nos.1&2.

## Part Four

This is the first time either of these papers have been published.

## Part Five

'Linking lives around shared themes: Narrative group therapy with gay men' by Christopher Behan was first published in *Gecko,* 1999 No.2.

'Weaving new stories over the phone: A narrative approach to a Gay Switchboard' by Bill Logan, as well as the following reflections, were first published in *Gecko,* 1999 No.3.

## Part Six

These three papers were first published in *Dulwich Centre Journal,* 1999 No.1.

## Part Seven

'Gender belonging: children, adolescents, adults and the role of the therapist; by Esben Esther Pirelli Benestad was first published in *Gecko,* 2001 No.1.

'About the expected expert' by *Mercedes Martinez*, and 'A reflection from a transgender perspective' by Esben Esther Pirelli Benestad were first published in *Gecko,* 2000 No.3.

## Part Eight

This is the first time any of these papers or interviews have been published, except for 'Who am I? Who are my people? And where do I belong?' by Claire Ralfs which was first published in *Dulwich Centre Journal,* 2000 Nos.1&2.

# References

Adams, A., Doering, R.W., Mitchell, J.N. & Wild, J. 1999: *Archives of Sexual Behavior*, 2.

Alcoff, L. & Gray, L. 1993: 'Survivor discourse: Transgression or recuperation?' *Signs: Journal of women in culture and society*, 18(2):260-290, Winter. University of Chicago Press.

Almås, E. & Benestad, E. 1999: 'Ord og begreper om kjønn, kjønnstilhørighet, kjønnsidentitet og seksuell orientering.' (Words and concepts about sex, gender, gender belonging, gender identity and sexual orientation.) *Impuls*, 3.

Almås, E. & Benestad, E. 1997: 'Væren i Systemene.' (Being in systems.) *Fokus på Familien*, 3-4:207-221.

Althusser, L. 1971: 'Ideology and ideological state apparatuses.' *Lenin and Philosophy*.

Armstrong, E. 1995: 'Traitors to the cause? Understanding the lesbian/gay "bisexuality debates".' In Tucker, N. with Highleyman, L. & Kaplan, R. (eds), *Bisexual Politics: Theories, queries & visions*, pp.199-217. Binghamton: Harrington Park Press.

Benestad, E.E.P. 2001: 'Gender belonging: Children, adolescents, adults and the role of the therapist.' *Gecko,* No.1.

Benestad, E. & Almås, E. 1993: 'Bekreftelsesmodell for kjønnstilhørighet.' (Confirmation model for gender belonging.) *Nordisk Sexologi*, 4:209-216.

Benestad, E.E.P. & Almaas, E. 2001: 'Kjoenn i bevegelse.' (Transforming gender.) *Univeritetsforlaget*, Oslo.

Bennett, K. 1992: 'Feminist bisexuality: A both/and option for an either/or world.' In Weise, E.R. (ed), *Closer to Home: Bisexuality and feminism.* Seattle, WA: Seal Press.

Bird, J. 2000: *The Heart's Narrative: Therapy and navigating life's contradictions.* Auckland: Edge Press.

Blanchard, R. & Steiner, B.W. 1990: *Clinical Management of Gender Identity Disorders in Children and Adults.* Washington, DC; London, England : American Psychiatric Press, Inc.

Blasingame, B.M. 1992: 'The roots of biphobia: Racism and internalized heterosexism.' In Weise, E.R. (ed), *Closer to Home: Bisexuality and Feminism.* Seattle: Seal Press.

Bornstein, K. 1994: *Gender Outlaw: On men, women, and the rest of us.* New York and London: Routledge.

Bornstein, K. 1995: *Gender Outlaw.* New York: Vintage Books.

Bradley, S.J, & Zucker, K.J. 1997: 'Gender identity disorder: A review of the past 10 years.' *J.Am. acad. child adolescent: psychiatry*, 36:7.

Card, C. 1992: 'Lesbianism and choice.' *Journal of Homosexuality*, 23(3):39-51.

Carrier J.M. 1986: 'Childhood cross-gender behavior and adult homosexuality.' *Archives of Sexual Behavior*, 15(1).

Carter, L. 1996: 'Sunday Mowing.' In C. McLean, M. Carey & C. White (eds), *Men's Ways of Being*, pp.135-144. Boulder, CO: Westview Press.

Cherubin, M., Flynn, W. & Morgan, A. 1998: 'Towards power and change: working with women carers in the mental health system.' *Gecko,* Vol 2.

Clark, D. 1977: *Loving Someone Gay.* Millbrae, CA: Celestial Arts.

Colker, R. 1996: *Hybrid: Bisexuals, multiracials, and other misfits under American law.* New York: New York University Press.

Combahee River Collective, 1981: 'A black feminist statement.' In Moraga, C. & Anzaldua, G. (eds), *This Bridge Called My Back: Writings by radical women of color,* pp.210-218. New York: Kitchen Table: Women of Color Press.

Davies, N. et al. 1996: *PINK Therapy.* Buckingham, Philadelphia: Open University Press.

Diamond, M. & Sigmundsson, H.K. 1997: 'Sex reassignment at birth. Long-term review and clinical implications.' *Arch. Pediatr.Adolesc.Med*, Vol.151, March.

Donaldson, S. 1995: 'The bisexual movement's beginnings in the 70s: A personal retrospective.' In Tucker, N. with Highleyman, L. & Kaplan, R. (eds), *Bisexual Politics: Theories, queries & visions*, pp.31-45. Binghamton: Harrington Park Press.

Doorn, D.C. 1997: 'Towards a Gender Identity Theory of Transsexualism.' Dissertation, Vrije Universiteit, Academisch Proefschrift, Amsterdam.

Doorn, C., Gooren L., Cohen-Kettenis, P., Verschoor A. & Kuiper A. Megens J. 1995: 'The processes of appraisal and self-verification in transsexualism and some of the consequences.' Presentasjon ved XIV Harry Benjamin International Gender Dysphoria Symposium, Kloster Irsee, Bayern, Tyskland, 7-10 September.

DSM-IV. Diagnostic and Statistical Manual of Mental Disorders, Forth Edition. The American Psychiatric Association, Washington , DC 1994.

Fekaris, D. & Perren, F. 1978: *I Will Survive.* Polygram International Publishing.

Firestein, B.A. 1996: 'Bisexuality as paradigm shift: Transforming our disciplines.' In Firestein, B.A. (ed), *Bisexuality: The psychology and politics of an invisible minority*, pp.263-291. Thousand Oaks, CA: Sage Publications.

Foucault, M. 1979: *Discipline and Punish: The birth of the prison. Trans. Alan Sheridan.* New York: Random House.

Foucault, M. 1990: *The History of Sexuality: An introduction (Vol.I). Trans. Robert Hurley.* New York: Vintage.

Garber, M. 1995: *Vice Versa: Bisexuality and the eroticism of everyday life*. New York: Simon & Schuster.

Gay Revolution Party Women's Caucus, 1972: 'Realesbians and Politicalesbians.' In Jay, K. & Young, A. (eds), *Out of the Closets: Voices of gay liberation.* New York: Douglas Book Corp.

Gilfus, M., 1999: 'The price of the ticket.' *Signs: Journal of women in culture and society*. University of Chicago Press.

Godden, R. 1991: *In This House of Brede.* (film) Amereon Ltd.

Gooren L., Delemarre-van de Waal, H. 1996: 'The feasibility of endocrine interventions in juvenile transsexuals.' *Journal of Psychology & Human Sexuality*, 8(4).

Green, R. 1968: 'Childhood cross- gender identification.' *Journal of Nervous and Mental Diseases*, 147:500-509.

Green, R. 1974: *Sexual identity conflict in children and adults*. New York: Basic Books

Green, R. 1987: *The 'Sissy Boy Syndrome' and the Development of Homosexuality*. New Haven, CT: Yale University Press.

Hegna, K., Kristiansen, H.W. & Moseng, B.U. 1999: 'Levekår og livskvalitet blant lesbiske kvinner og homofile menn.' (Livings conditions and quality of life among lesbian women and homosexual men.) *NOVA*, Oslo, p.320-321.

Hoffman, L. 1998: 'Family therapy: A braided challah.' Paper presented at the conference of the Texas Association of Marriage and Family Therapists, Dallas, Texas.

hooks, b. 1984: *Feminist Theory: From margin to center*. Boston: South End Press.

Jordan, J. 1994: 'A new politics of sexuality.' *Technical Difficulties*. New York: Vintage.

Ka'ahumanu, L. 1995: 'It ain't over 'til the bisexual speaks.' In Tucker, N. with Highleyman, L. & Kaplan, R. (eds), *Bisexual Politics: Theories, queries & visions*, pp.63-68. Binghamton: Harrington Park Press.

Kaplan, R. 1992: 'Compulsory heterosexuality and bisexual existence: Toward a bisexual feminist understanding of heterosexism.' In Weise, E.R. (ed), *Closer to Home: Bisexuality and feminism*, pp.269-280. Seattle: Seal Press.

Keratin, J. 1988: 'Lesbian daughters and lesbian mothers: The crisis of disclosure from a family systems perspective.' In Braverman, L. (ed), *A Guide to Feminist Family Therapy*. NY: Harrington Park Press.

Kermode, F. 1966: *The Sense of an Ending: Studies in the theory of fiction*. New York & London: Oxford University Press.

Kessler, S.J. & McKenna, W. 1978: *Gender: An ethnomethodological approach*. New York: John Wiley & Sons.

Kitzinger, C. & Perkins, R. 1993: *Changing Our Minds: Lesbian feminism and psychology*. New York University.

Kivel, P. 1996: *Uprooting racism: How white people can work for racial justice*. Gabriola Island, BC, Canada: New Society Publishers.

Madigan, S. & Epston, D. 1995: 'From "Spy-chiatric" Gaze to Communities of Concern: From professional monologue to dialogue.' In Friedman, S. (ed), *The Reflecting Team in Action: Collaborative practice in family therapy*, pp.257-276. New York: Guilford Publications.

Martin, B. 1988: 'Lesbian identity and autobiographical difference[s].' In Brodski, B. & Schenck, C. (eds), *Life/Lines: Theorizing women's autobiography.* Ithaca and London: Cornell University Press.

Martin, B. & Mohanty, C.T. 1986: 'Feminist politics: What's home got to do with it?' In deLauretis, T. (ed), *Feminist Studies/Critical Studies*, pp.191-212. Bloomington: Indiana University Press.

Mayne, J. 1991: 'Lesbian looks: Dorothy Arzner and female authorship.' In Bad Object Choices (ed), *How Do I Look?* Queer Film and Video, pp.103-135. Seattle: Bay Press.

McKeon, E. 1992: 'To be bisexual and underclass.' In Weise, E.R. (ed), *Closer to Home: Bisexuality and feminism.* Seattle, WA: Seal Press.

Miller, D.A. 1981: *Narrative and Its Discontents: Problems of closure in the traditional novel.* Princeton: Princeton University Press.

Moraga, C. 1981: 'La Guera.' *This Bridge Called My Back: Writings By radical women of color*, pp.27-34. New York: Kitchen Table: Women of Color Press.

Morris, J. 1997: *Conundrum.* London: Penguin Books.

Moss, P & Butterworth, P. 1999: 'Introducing mosaic.' In *Narrative Therapy and Community Work: A conference collection.* Adelaide: Dulwich Centre Publications.

Myerhoff, B. 1978: *Number Our Days.* New York: Simon and Shuster.

Neilsen, J. 1988-92: 'The power of the language we use.' *Out/Look,* Fall.

Nossel, M., 1999: 'The story-telling group.' *Dulwich Centre Journal*, No.3.

Ochs, R. 1996: 'Biphobia: It goes more than two ways.' In Firestein, B.A. (ed), *Bisexuality: The psychology and politics of an invisible minority.* Thousand Oaks, CA: Sage.

O'Keefe, T. & Fox, K. 1997: *TRANS-X-U-ALL, The naked Difference.* London: Extraordinary People Press.

Pramaggiore, M. 1996: 'Straddling the screen: Bisexual spectatorship and contemporary narrative film.' In Hall, D.E. & Pramaggiore, M. (eds), *RePresenting BiSexualities: Subjects and cultures of fluid desire*, PP.272-297. New York & London: New York University Press.

Pratt, M.B. 1984: 'Identity: Skin blood heart.' In Bulkin, E. et al. (eds), *Yours In Struggle: Three feminist perspectives on anti-Semitism and racism*, pp.9-63. Brooklyn, New York: Long Haul Press.

Rich, A. 1980: 'Compulsory heterosexuality and lesbian existence.' *Signs*, 5:631-660 (Summer).

Rich, A. 1993: 'Compulsory heterosexuality and lesbian existence.' In *Blood, Bread, and Poetry, Selected Prose 1979-1985.* Reprinted in Richardson, L. & Taylor, V. (eds), *Feminist Frontiers III*, pp.158-179. New York: McGraw-Hill.

Rodgers, N. & Edwards, B. 1979: *We Are Family.* Atlantic Recording.

Rust, P. 1995: *Bisexuality and the Challenge to Lesbian Politics: Sex, loyalty, and revolution.* New York: New York University Press.

Schroder, M. 1997: University of Chicago: New Woman´s Gynecological Index, presentation on The 2nd International Congress on Sex & Gender Issues, King of Preussia, PA; Juna 19-22.

Shuster, R. (1992): 'Bisexuality and the quest for principled loving.' In Weise, E.R. (ed), *Closer to Home: Bisexuality and feminism.* Seattle, WA: Seal Press.

Sisters Inside can be contacted at www.sistersinside.com.au

Som, Indigo Chih-Lien, 1995: 'The queer kitchen.' In The Bisexual Anthology Collective (eds), *Plural Desires: Writing bisexual women's realities*, pp.84-88. Toronto: Sister Vision.

Stacey, K. 1993: 'Exploring stories of lesbian experience in therapy: Implications for therapists in a postmodern world.' *Dulwich Centre Newsletter,* No.2

Stoller R.J. 1965: 'The sense of maleness.' *Psychoanalytic Quarterly*, 34:207-218.

Stoller R.J. 1968: 'The sense of femaleness.' *Psychoanalytic Quarterly*, 37:42-55.

Sullivan, C., Lowry, B., Bradly, S.J. & Zucker, K.J 1995: Chapter 17 in Vincent B.Van Hasselt & Michel Hersen (eds), *Handbook of Adolescent Psychopathology.* New York, London, Toronto, Sydney, Tokyo, Singapore: Lexington Books.

The Harry Benjamins International Gender Dysphoria Association 2001: 'The Standards of Care for Gender Identity Disorders – sixth version.' *The International Journal of Transgenderism*, 5(1),January-March.

Trudinger, M., Boyd, C. & Melrose, P. 1998: 'Questioning sexuality: A workshop in progress.' *Dulwich Centre Journal*, No.4. 'Working on issues of violence and abuse' (special issue).

Udis-Kessler, A. 1995: 'Identity/politics: A history of the bisexual movement.' In Tucker, N. with Highleyman, L. & Kaplan, R. (eds), *Bisexual Politics: Theories, queries & visions*, pp.17-30. Binghamton: Harrington Park Press.

Van der Ven, A. 1998. 'A visual model for transgenderism as a process of self-discovery' or 'Who would you like to be in two years?' Presentation on The third International Congress of Sex and Gender, Oxford, 18-20 September.

Welch, S.D. 1990: *A Feminist Ethic of Risk*. Minneapolis, MN: Fortress Press.

White, M. 1995: 'Reflecting teamwork as definitional ceremony.' In White, M., *Re-Authoring Lives: Interviews and Essays*. Adelaide: Dulwich Centre Publications.

White M. 1995: 'The politics of therapy' (chapter 2) and 'Outside expert knowledge' (chapter 3). *Re-Authoring Lives: Interviews & essays*. Adelaide: Dulwich Centre Publications.

White, M. 1997: *Narratives of Therapist's Lives*. Adelaide: Dulwich Centre Publications.

Wingard, B. & Lester, J, 2001: *Telling our stories in ways that make us stronger*. Adelaide: Dulwich Centre Publications.

Women and Mental Health Inc can be contacted on wamhnsw@netspace.net.au
Copies of the report 'Every Boundary Broken' can be ordered via the WAMH email.

Yalom, I.D. 1985: *Theory and Practice of Group Psychotherapy*. New York: Basic Books.

Zucker, K.J., Bradley, S.J., Kuksis, M., Pecore, K., Birkenfeld-Adams, A., Doering, R.W., Mitchell, J.N. & Wild, J. 1999: 'Gender constancy judgments in children with gender identity disorder: Evidence for developmental lag.' *Archives of Sexual Behaviour*, 2.